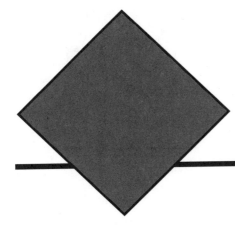

Examination Preparation

A Complete Guide
for the Physical Therapist

Scott M. Giles M.S., P.T.

Clinical Associate Professor
Department of Physical Therapy
University of New England
Biddeford, Maine

Ronda Sanders M.Ed., C.E.T.

Assistant Professor
Department of Learning Assistance and Individual Learning
University of New England
Biddeford, Maine

MT

Mainely Physical Therapy
P.O. Box 7242
Scarborough, Maine 04070-7242

Toll Free: (866) PTEXAMS
Phone: (207) 885-0304
Fax: (207) 883-8377
Web site: www.ptexams.com

3/21/04

Acknowledgments

My sincere thanks to Therese Giles
and Gwenn Hoyt for their
valuable assistance with this project

Love to Traci, Meghan, Erin, Alexander, and Zachary

Special thanks to the many students who have
served as a constant source of inspiration

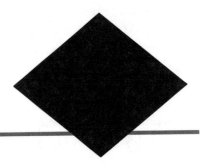

Table of Contents

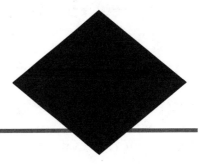

Introduction

The word examination can strike fear and anxiety into individuals like few other words in the English language. What is it about an examination that is so threatening to the majority of the population? The American Heritage Dictionary defines the word examination as "a set of questions designed to test knowledge." Although students are frequently exposed to examinations throughout their academic training, the thought of a comprehensive examination can make even the sturdiest student begin to perspire.

In physical therapy, the ultimate comprehensive examination is the Physical Therapist Examination. The national examination serves to measure the knowledge and skills necessary for minimal competency in the field of physical therapy and is often the final hurdle a physical therapist must clear before obtaining licensure.

Perhaps a candidate's apprehension can be more clearly understood when viewing the significance of this examination. Candidates, in most cases, have recently completed their academic preparation and are eager to embark on their professional careers. They recognize that failure to meet or exceed the minimum scoring requirement on the examination can act as a barrier prohibiting them from practicing as an independent professional.

Our text is designed to maximize a candidate's performance on the Physical Therapist Examination. The text will accomplish this goal by taking candidates through eight distinct and separate units.

Unit One: Physical Therapist Examination
Unit One provides indepth information on the Physical Therapist Examination. It outlines the purpose, format, and design of the examination and addresses issues ranging from registration to scoring.

Unit Two: Time Management
Unit Two allows candidates to assess their time management skills. Candidates are presented with useful guidelines to consider when designing a study schedule.

Unit Three: You as a Learner

Unit Three provides candidates with the opportunity to assess their individual learning style. Candidates are shown how this information can be utilized as they prepare for the Physical Therapist Examination.

Unit Four: Study Plan

Unit Four explores the many different components of an effective study plan. Candidates are presented with valuable information to guide them as they develop an individualized study plan.

Unit Five: Multiple Choice Examinations

Unit Five analyzes the various components of a multiple choice examination. Suggested techniques to assist candidates when analyzing multiple choice questions are introduced. Candidates are given the opportunity to refine their test taking skills by answering selected examination questions.

Unit Six: Content Outline

Unit Six provides candidates with the opportunity to explore the content outline of the Physical Therapist Examination. A summary of each of the categories within the content outline is provided along with selected sample questions.

Unit Seven: Final Preparation

Unit Seven discusses issues for candidates to consider on the final days prior to the Physical Therapist Examination. Specific strategies to maximize performance and limit anxiety are discussed.

Unit Eight: Sample Examination

Unit Eight consists of a sample 200 question examination. Candidates are given the opportunity to refine their test taking skills and to assess their level of preparedness for the actual examination.

Physical Therapist Examination

The Physical Therapist Examination is a 225 question, multiple choice examination. The examination is designed to determine if candidates possess the minimal competency necessary to practice as physical therapists.

The examination is created under the auspices of the Federation of State Boards of Physical Therapy. According to the National Physical Therapy Examination Candidate Handbook, the examination program serves two important purposes:

1. Provide examination services to authorities charged with the regulation of physical therapists and physical therapist assistants.

2. Provide a common element in evaluation of candidates so that standards will be comparable from jurisdiction to jurisdiction.

Registration

Registration occurs at the state level through the Physical Therapy State Licensing Agencies. The address of each agency, phone number, and web site are provided in the Appendix. Some state licensing agencies now permit online registration through the Federation of State Boards of Physical Therapy. Eligibility requirements vary considerably from jurisdiction to jurisdiction; therefore it is imperative that candidates carefully read all application information.

A variety of items may be required as part of the application process. These items may include a photograph; a notarized birth certificate; an official transcript from an accredited school; professional reference letters; and a check or money order for the required application, examination, and licensing fees.

It cannot be emphasized enough, however, that individual state licensing agencies' requirements vary. One small example is that many states will not accept any form of payment other than a money order or a certified bank check. If an applicant uses another form of payment, such as a personal check, the application could be considered incomplete. To avoid such difficulties, it is prudent to read the application carefully and to inquire as to the status of the application approximately two weeks after the completed application has been submitted.

Some states offer candidates with verifiable employment the opportunity to practice prior to being licensed by issuing a temporary license. Typically, candidates are required to have a completed application on file and have met all other qualifications for licensure before being considered for the temporary license. Temporary licenses are usually revoked if a candidate receives notification he/she was not successful on the Physical Therapist Examination.

Licensure

There are two primary ways in which to obtain a license to practice as a physical therapist. They are termed examination and endorsement.

Examination
Licensure by examination is obtained after a candidate meets or exceeds the minimum scoring requirement on the Physical Therapist Examination and has satisfied all other state requirements. This form of obtaining licensure is the traditional method for candidates seeking initial licensure.

Endorsement
Licensure by endorsement using the Federation of State Boards of Physical Therapy Score Transfer Service makes it possible for candidates who have been licensed in a state by virtue of an examination to potentially gain licensure in another state without retaking the examination. Examination scores can be transferred to any physical therapy state licensing agency via the Federation of State Boards of Physical Therapy Score Transfer Service. The web site address for the Federation of State Boards of Physical Therapy is available in the Appendix.

Foreign Trained Therapists
Foreign trained therapists are often subjected to a myriad of requirements before they are eligible to become licensed in the United States. Since the requirements vary significantly by state, it is recommended that candidates contact the physical therapy state licensing agency within the state they intend to practice. The state licensing agency can provide detailed information on their individual requirements.

There are two general requirements which seem to be consistent in all states for foreign trained therapists:

1. Applicants are required to submit their educational credentials for evaluation of their equivalence to the United States trained applicant.

2. Applicants must meet or exceed the minimum scoring requirement on the Physical Therapist Examination.

Other state requirements can include, but are not limited to, the following:

- Demonstrate proficiency in written and spoken English
- Submit letters of reference
- Obtain a valid visa and resident alien card
- Complete an internship or period of supervised practice
- Appear for an interview
- Attain the equivalent of a United States grade of "C" or higher in all professional coursework

Examination Development

According to the Federation of State Boards of Physical Therapy, the Physical Therapist Examination is developed by three committees. These committees are the Examination Construction and Review Committee; the Item Bank Review Committee; and the Item Writer Regional Coordinators.

The Examination Construction and Review Committee is responsible for determining the content categories and subcategories of the examination and the percentage of items in each area. The categories are based on the tasks and roles that comprise the practice of physical therapy. The information necessary to create each category and subcategory is obtained after analyzing the responses of hundreds of physical therapists to a job analysis survey. The most recent job analysis survey occurred in 2001 and was introduced in the new content outline in November of 2002. The content outline is typically revised on a five year cycle.

Individual physical therapists have direct involvement in the writing of examination questions. The physical therapists involved are required to attend item-writing workshops that are taught by experienced testing professionals. Questions, once completed, are analyzed independently to make sure they are reflective of the current examination content outline. The focus of the examination questions is on problem solving and away from rote memorization of fact. Candidates are required to demonstrate their ability to apply knowledge in a safe and effective manner.

Examination Administration

Candidates begin the application process by obtaining a general application form and a computerized scannable information form from a physical therapy state licensing agency. Once completed, the forms are returned along with any necessary fees to the state licensing agency. After a candidate's application is approved, the state licensing agency forwards the computerized form to the Federation of State Boards of Physical Therapy. A limited number of states are now permitting candidates to apply online through the Federation of State Boards of Physical Therapy.

The Federation of State Boards of Physical Therapy issues candidates an "approval to test" letter that includes instructions on how to schedule an appointment to take the examination. Candidates must sit for the examination within 60 days of the date on their letter. The examination is offered on computer at over 300 Prometric Testing Centers within the United States or at selected testing facilities in Canada. Testing is offered Monday through Saturday from 9:00 AM - 6:00 PM. Within each Prometric Testing Center candidates can concentrate on the examination without environmental distracters. Private, modular booths provide adequate work space with proper lighting and ventilation. All Prometric Testing Centers are fully accessible.

Candidates are not limited to the testing centers within the state they are applying for licensure. For example, a student that has recently graduated from a physical therapy program in Maine could apply for licensure in California and take the required examination while still in Maine.

It is important to note that basic computer skills are not necessary with computer based testing. Prior to beginning the examination, candidates utilize a tutorial which explains topics such as selecting answers and navigating within the examination. Time spent on the computer tutorial does not count towards the allotted time for the actual examination.

Candidates have the option of entering their answers using a computer keyboard or mouse. Once within the actual examination candidates can move freely between examination questions. Candidates can go back to previously answered or unanswered questions and make any desired changes. Candidates are allowed to use scratch paper supplied by the testing center during the examination.

Content Outline

The content outline provides candidates with a detailed description of the information contained on the Physical Therapist Examination. Although listed here, the content outline will be discussed in detail in Unit Six.

Physical Therapist Examination

I. Examination
History and Systems Review

Tests and Measures Group I
1. Strength, ROM, Posture, Body Structures, Prosthetic & Orthotic Devices
2. Cognition, Nerve, Reflex and Sensory Integrity, Neurodevelopment

Tests and Measures Group II
1. Cardiovascular/pulmonary System
2. Integumentary System

II. Evaluation, Diagnosis, Prognosis, and Outcomes
Evaluation and Diagnosis
Prognosis and Outcomes

III. Intervention
Non-procedural Intervention
1. Coordination of care
2. Communication
3. Documentation
4. Patient/family/client-related instructions

Procedural Intervention
Group I: Exercise and manual therapy

Group II: Transfer and functional activities, gait training, assistive and adaptive devices, and modification of the environment

Group III: Physical agents and modalities, airway clearance techniques, wound care, and promoting health and wellness

IV. Standards of Care
1. Maintaining patient autonomy, confidentiality, and obtaining informed consent
2. Recognizing scope of physical therapy practice, including limitations of the PT role that necessitate referral to other disciplines
3. Utilizing body mechanics/positioning
4. Considering the patient's cultural background, social history, home situation, and geographic barriers, etc.
5. Safety, CPR, emergency care, first aid, standard precautions

Scoring

The actual Physical Therapist Examination is 225 questions, however 25 of the questions serve as pretest items and are not officially scored. The pretest items allow new examination questions to be evaluated throughout the year and eliminate lengthy delays in score reporting. Candidates are unable to differentiate between pretest and scored items on the 225 question examination. To accommodate for the increased number of questions, candidates receive an additional 30 minutes to complete the examination. Candidates have a total of 4.5 hours to complete the 225 question examination. Since candidate performance is based solely on the number of scored items answered correctly, the sample examination in Unit Eight consists of only 200 questions.

The Federation of State Boards of Physical Therapy is responsible for scoring the examination and reporting results to the individual state licensing agencies. The state licensing agencies then notify candidates as to their performance on the examination. Formal notification typically occurs through the mail, however many state licensing agencies have web sites that allow candidates to determine their licensing status online. In most instances, candidates' scores are available within 3-10 days.

The questions are multiple choice with four possible answers to each question. Candidates are asked to identify the best answer to each of the questions. Each question has only one correct answer. A candidate's score is determined based on the number of questions answered correctly. Candidates accumulate one point for each correctly answered question. There is no penalty for questions answered incorrectly. The total cumulative score is termed the total raw score. The maximum total raw score for the Physical Therapist Examination is 200.

Criterion-referenced scoring is used to determine passing scores on the Physical Therapist Examination. Passing scores are determined based on the judgment of selected experts on the minimum number of questions that should be answered correctly by a minimally qualified candidate. Criterion-referenced passing scores are determined independently of candidate performance and are designed to reflect the difficulty of each examination. For example, if a given examination was judged to be particularly difficult, the minimum passing score would be lower than another examination that was judged to be less difficult.

Since the minimum passing score is based on the difficulty of the examination, it becomes impossible to determine an automatic passing score. Historically, criterion-referenced passing scores have ranged from 135 - 152. If the criterion-referenced passing score was established as 144 for a given examination, a total raw score of greater than or equal to 144 would be considered a passing score, while a total raw score of less than 144 would be considered a failing score. Within a given examination cycle, criterion-referenced passing scores usually fluctuate in a much smaller range, perhaps by as few as five questions.

An individual examination score is often reported to candidates in the form of a scaled score. Scaled scores range from 200 - 800 with the minimum passing score always being equal to a scaled score of 600. Scaled scores are necessary as a method of equating examinations with different criterion-referenced passing scores.

If a candidate is successful on the examination, in most cases they have fulfilled the final requirement for licensure. Conversely, if a candidate is unsuccessful on the examination, he/she is required to reapply to the state licensing agency. With computer based testing there is no mandatory waiting period before retaking the examination, however some states limit the number of times a candidate can take the examination or mandate remedial coursework.

Candidates that were unsuccessful on the Physical Therapist Examination can elect to receive role feedback. The role feedback report compares individual examination performance with that of other candidates taking the same examination. Additional information on role feedback is available through the Federation of State Boards of Physical Therapy.

In addition to the Physical Therapist Examination, a number of states also require candidates to successfully complete a jurisprudence examination. This type of examination is based on the state rules and regulations governing physical therapy practice. The examination can include multiple choice items, short answer questions, or fill in the blanks. States can administer the examination using computer based testing or even as a take home examination.

Coming Attractions

As you have progressed through this unit, you most likely have gained an appreciation for the complexity of preparing for the Physical Therapist Examination. Although this task can, at times, seem overwhelming there are a number of strategies that can significantly enhance a candidate's preparation efficiency and organization. These areas are:

- Time management skills
- A viable study plan
- Knowledge of how you learn
- Test taking skills

Each of these four areas will be discussed in detail in upcoming units. Candidates should attempt to apply the information obtained in these units as they prepare for the Physical Therapist Examination.

Time Management

Time management is, perhaps, the most overlooked component of a comprehensive study plan. Most candidates take the Physical Therapist Examination shortly after graduation. This can be a very anxious and unsettled time. Candidates often are actively seeking employment or are attempting to adjust to a new job. They may have relocated to a different residence or perhaps moved to another part of the country. To further complicate matters, they are starting to focus on the impending Physical Therapist Examination.

Time Management Assessment

Time management is not about meeting deadlines and getting things done. Time management is about keeping our lives in balance. We will classify the major areas of our lives into four distinct and separate categories. These areas are listed and defined below:

The emotional you: your inner self - your ongoing and ever-changing perceptions and reflections on life, self, values, etc.

The intellectual you: your intellectually curious self - student, reader, researcher, etc.

The physical you: your physical self - walking, running, swimming, grooming, etc.

The social you: your outer self - social interactions with family, friends, church activities, etc.

When the balance among these four areas is disturbed, stress inevitably results. One of the major by-products of stress is the inability to concentrate and retain information. Failure to concentrate while preparing for a comprehensive examination such as the Physical Therapist Examination can have devastating results.

How balanced are your days? Find out by keeping an Activity Log for a three day period. A sample Activity Log is located in the Appendix. Attempt to follow your normal daily routine during these three days. At the end of each day, summarize your activity using the Time Management Diagnostic Sheet.

Time Management Diagnostic Sheet

	Day One	Day Two	Day Three	Total
CLASS				
STUDY				
INDIVIDUAL TIME				
SOCIAL TIME				
EXERCISE				
WORK				
SLEEP				
NAP				
NIGHT				
SPECIAL APPOINTMENT				

After completing the diagnostic activity sheet, attempt to determine how balanced your days are. Ask yourself if there are any of the four areas of your life that are not represented in your daily activities. If deficient areas are identified, attempt to select activities to augment these areas.

Are you getting some physical activity? A twenty minute walk may be sufficient. Did you find time, or did you simply not get around to it? Was it too cold out, or did you simply not feel like exercising?

How about your social self? These times include social functions, conversations with friends and family, or non-working lunches. Did you avoid others because you were not feeling very sociable, or did you feel you had too much to do without wasting time playing?

Did you nurture your emotional self? This reflective area of life is the most diverse among people, and often the most neglected. Some people serve their emotional needs in church, some like to meditate or listen to music. Did you avoid such activities because you felt you simply did not have the time to spare or did you feel it was relatively unimportant with all of your other pressing needs?

How about intellectual stimulation? Probably at this point your intellectual self is being pandered to for many hours each day preparing for the examination. However, it is healthy to have a few other intellectual pursuits not related to the examination. Have you placed other intellectual pursuits like reading the newspaper or watching the news on hold because you are immersed in preparing for the examination with every waking moment?

Candidates also need to assess their ability to concentrate. Do you find yourself drifting off and glancing at the clock to discover that twenty minutes has elapsed and you have no idea where the time went? Do you feel that your study breaks seem to get longer as your study session progresses? Do you elect not to take study breaks and find yourself waking up in the cold, early hours of the morning, slumped over your books with a sore neck? Can you find a million "necessary" chores to do in order to avoid settling down to study?

If you answered yes to any of the preceding questions, you may benefit from improved time management. Remember, stress is progressive, so the ability to concentrate and retain information will decrease as time goes on. We suggest that you try the following two-part program.

Time Management Program

Part One: Long-Range Planning

Step 1: Find a calendar and identify the months between now and when you plan to take the examination.

Step 2: Use the content outline and begin to assign time to each of the four content areas so that they can be reviewed adequately prior to the examination.

Since the four content areas vary significantly in their weighting, it is imperative that candidates also weight the study time dedicated to each area. The specific weighting of each of the content areas is discussed in detail in Unit Six.

A sample two-month, long-range schedule is illustrated below:

Sample Two Month Long-Range Schedule

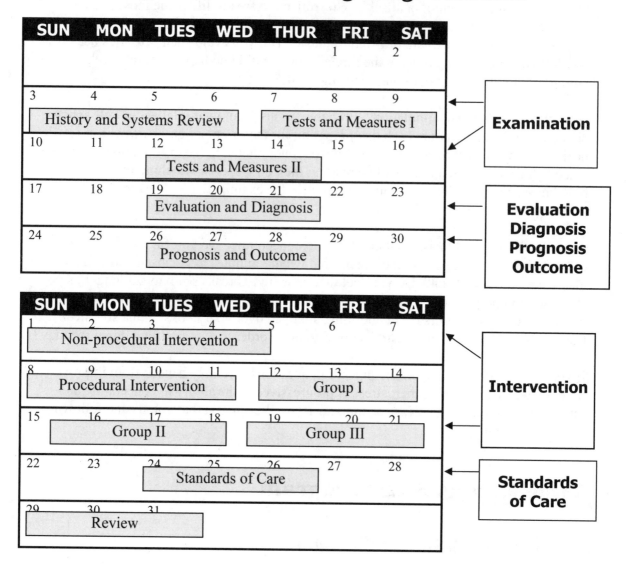

Part Two: Weekly Planning

Step 1:   Assign a color to each of the four areas of your life: emotional, intellectual, physical, and social.

Step 2:   Develop a master weekly schedule that includes all of your scheduled activities. These activities can include items such as: study sessions, work, church, social engagements and exercise sessions. Mark each of the activities that appear on the master schedule with the appropriate color.

Step 3:   Determine which, if any, of the four areas is being neglected in your present schedule. Select activities that can augment the deficient areas and assign them times, keeping in mind the following:

    Emotional: Individual reflection time allocated for thinking about issues important to you; done independently, goal-directed, resolution-oriented, time-limited; most people plan for one half-hour, or two fifteen minute periods daily, neither just before bed.

    Intellectual: Involves study time or clinical practice; follow the study plan suggested for your learning style, taking into consideration your learning environment preferences (Unit Three).

    Physical: Works best if not done immediately after a meal or just before bedtime; combines well with emotional or social time immediately afterwards.

    Social: Includes meal time, movies, theater, etc; works best when scheduled before a firm commitment, since individuals are most likely to lose track of time in this area.

Step 4:   Complete the schedule, being sure to leave at least one hour each day unfilled. When a scheduled activity is missed, it can be rescheduled easily within the available time.

Step 5:   Follow the schedule for at least one week and then do a self-assessment of your satisfaction with your productivity and concentration during study times. You may find it necessary to make adjustments to your future schedule based on your progress.

The following table illustrates a sample weekly schedule, which has been coded to correspond to each of the four areas of your life. By quickly examining the schedule, it becomes fairly easy to determine the relative weighting of each area. Candidates should attempt to design an individual schedule that is consistent with their present life status.

Sample Weekly Time Management Schedule

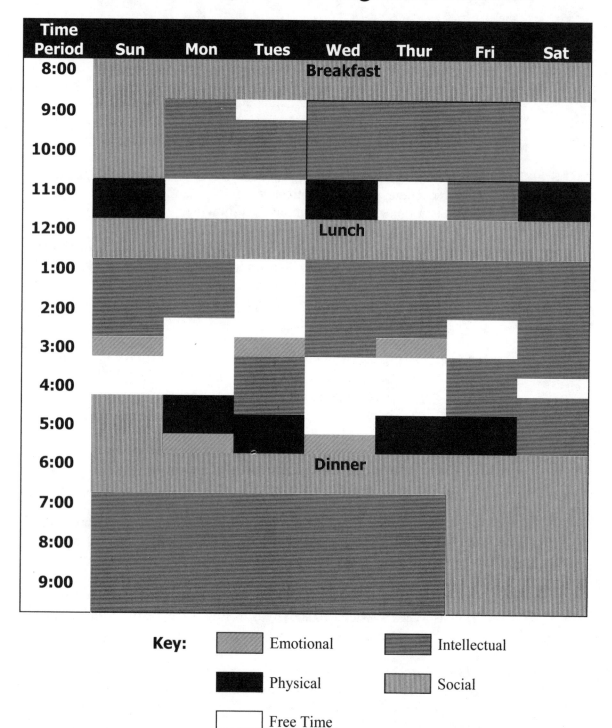

Time Period	Sun	Mon	Tues	Wed	Thur	Fri	Sat
8:00				Breakfast			
9:00							
10:00							
11:00							
12:00				Lunch			
1:00							
2:00							
3:00							
4:00							
5:00							
6:00				Dinner			
7:00							
8:00							
9:00							

Key:
- Emotional
- Intellectual
- Physical
- Social
- Free Time

You as a Learner

We imagine that at some time during your college years, you have observed the most obnoxious learner of all, the one who never seems to study and then consistently receives an "A" on every examination. This person does not necessarily have any more intelligence than other students, but simply may have developed a sense of how he/she learns most efficiently and is therefore able to develop a study plan based on his/her individual learning needs. It is our hope that the time management strategies presented earlier, in combination with the material that will be conveyed in this unit, will enable you to develop an efficient and effective individualized study plan.

To discover how you function as a learner, you need to answer three specific questions:

1. What combination of the three learning channels do you prefer for input and processing?
2. What is your dominant thinking mode?
3. What is your optimum learning environment?

The Three Learning Channels

There are three basic ways of perceiving information: see it (visual), hear it (auditory), or be physically involved in doing it (tactile/kinesthetic). The combination of these channels that an individual uses, both the first time he/she is exposed to new material (input) and during subsequent exposure (processing), determines one of the facets of learning style. Each individual's preference of channels for input and processing determines Active/Passive learning patterns.

Attempt to classify your preferred learning style for input and processing into one of the following four categories:

Active/Active

If you are an individual who, the first time you are exposed to new material likes to hear it, see it, say it, question it, interact with it, and then keep right on doing this, you would be categorized as a multisensoral (visual, auditory, and tactile/kinesthetic) active learner for both input and processing. These individuals immediately attempt to determine the relevance and utility of material and must, at input, be able to relate it to previous knowledge or experience. They typically find it difficult, and sometimes impossible, to go into a room alone, open up a book, and read.

Strengths:
- focus on application and utility of ideas
- 100% concentration on activities for short periods of time
- flexibility and adaptability

Weaknesses:
- may consider details boring
- short attention span may lead to incomplete preparation
- high distractibility may disrupt concentration

Active/Passive

If you are an individual who, the first time you are exposed to new material, likes to hear it, see it, say it, question it, interact with it, and then take a visual reference home to study by yourself, you would be classified as a multisensoral learner for input and a visual processor. These individuals need to relate new material, at input, to previous knowledge or experience.

Strengths:
- focus on gathering extensive data
- long-term memory
- strong visual channel often allows them to visualize notes, text, charts in their mind's eye

Weaknesses:
- may not focus on utility or use of information
- may require more time to learn new material
- may have a tendency to gather excessive information in an area of special interest and neglect other important areas

Passive/Active

If you are an individual who, the first time you are exposed to new material, likes either to hear it in lecture form or to read it in a book, and then utilize the material in an interactive way (visual, auditory, tactile/kinesthetic), you would be categorized as a passive learner for input and an active processor. These individuals relate new material to previous knowledge or experience and determine the relevance and utility of the material after input and before processing.

Strengths:

- focus on both facts/concepts and clinical application
- synthesis of known information into a plan of action
- sequential and relational thought

Weaknesses:

- may have difficulty determining proportional importance of information
- may begin applying information before sufficient details have been gathered
- may fail to identify the relationship to previous knowledge or experience

Passive/Passive

If you are an individual who, the first time you are exposed to new material, likes either to hear it or to read it and prefers to keep right on doing that, you would be categorized as a passive learner for both input and processing. These individuals determine the relationship to known material after input and before processing.

Strengths:

- sequential thinking
- focus on details
- strong visual channel that allows one to visualize notes, text, charts in their mind's eye

Weaknesses:

- may miss the "big picture"
- may have difficulty answering application questions requiring relational thinking
- tendency to study alone often inhibits opportunities to examine information from different perspectives

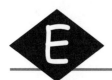

Exercise One

Once you have identified your preferred learning style for input and processing, attempt to classify the strength of your preference. We have divided this category into slight, decided and strong.

If all of the descriptors in one of the categories describe your learning style, place a check under strong preference. If the majority, but not all of the descriptors were accurate, place a check next to decided. If a few more of the descriptors in one category, when compared to the others, describe your learning style, place a check next to slight.

The stronger one's preference for a specific category, the less flexible a candidate will be in his/her input and processing channel needs. Candidates with a strong preference will need to pay particular attention to the recommendations for their learning style in Unit Four.

Input/Processing Preferences

	Slight	Decided	Strong
Active/Active	☐	☐	☐
Active/Passive	☐	☐	☐
Passive/Active	☐	☐	☐
Passive/Passive	☐	☐	☐
	◆	◆	◆

Thinking Modes

You probably have heard the terms "left-brained" and "right-brained." In this book, these are not physiological or psychological terms, but instead educational terms which describe a set of learning characteristics. The following table depicts "left-brain" and "right-brain" learners' characteristics:

"Left" Thinking	"Right" Thinking
Facts	"What if.....?"
Words	Pictures
Sequences	Relationships
Details	Global concepts
Analytical	Synthetic

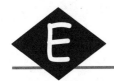

Exercise Two

Complete the following informal exercise to evaluate your thinking mode.

1. Look over the text and the chart. Both contain the same information. Assume you are attempting to learn the information for the first time and that you have no previous knowledge of fruits' shapes or colors.

    Fruits come in many shapes and colors. Oranges, kiwi, and tangerines are round; bananas are oblong; and pears are "pear shaped."

    Oranges and tangerines are orange; bananas and pears are yellow; a kiwi is green.

	Shape			Color		
	Round	Pear	Oblong	Orange	Yellow	Green
Oranges	•			•		
Tangerines	•			•		
Bananas			•		•	
Pears		•			•	
Kiwi	•					•

    If you were more comfortable learning the information about fruit from the two paragraphs of text, place an **X** next to the "L" below. If the table appealed to you more, place an **X** next to the "R". If you are equally comfortable with both, place an **X** next to the "I" (integrated).

    _____ "L"   _____ "I"   _____ "R"

2. Picture the following scenario: You are going downtown to do some errands. Your errands will require you to go to the bank, the post office, the hardware store, the gas station, and the grocery store. The location of each facility is as follows:

❖ **Bank**

❖ **Gas Station**

❖ **Grocery Store**

❖ **Hardware Store**

❖ **Post Office**

❖ **Your Home**

If, either before leaving the house or while you were driving, you would think about the sequence in which you plan to do the errands in the most efficient way, place an **X** next to the "L". If you would complete the errands in a random order, place an **X** next to the "R". If sometimes you would plan and sometimes you would not, place an **X** next to the "I".

_____ "L"   _____ "I"   _____ "R"

◆   ◆   ◆

Learning Environment

The following checklist, although by no means complete, can help you identify the learning environment best suited for your concentration and learning needs. Place a check mark in the boxes next to the items that you prefer.

Individual Preferences		
☐ Morning	☐ Afternoon	☐ Evening
☐ Quiet	☐ Soft Music	☐ Noisy
☐ Sitting	☐ Standing	☐ Moving
☐ Snacking	☐ Talking	☐ Writing
☐ Typing	☐ Colorful Room	☐ Muted Tones
☐ Alone	☐ Partner	☐ Group

Input/Processing Preferences			
Frequency of Meetings	☐ Regularly	☐ Often	☐ As Needed
Duration of Sessions	☐ One Hour	☐ Two Hours	☐ Flexible
Structure	☐ Hierarchical	☐ Participative	☐ Debate

Learning Profile Application

After progressing through the three learning style exercises, you may be wondering how this information can be utilized to assist you with your preparation for the Physical Therapist Examination. Each of the learning style activities provides unique insight into your individual learning style.

The knowledge acquired about your input and processing needs can be utilized as a guide to design your study schedule to suit your Active/Passive preferences. For example, if you have identified that you prefer to be active at input, you intentionally can incorporate visual, auditory, and/or tactile-kinesthetic stimulation into your study sessions. Let's assume that you are reviewing orthopedic special tests. The visual channel can be activated by reading orthopedic textbooks, examining pictures, or watching videotapes of selected special tests. The auditory channel can be activated by listening to yourself or others talk about selected special tests, and the tactile/kinesthetic channel can be utilized by performing selected special tests on another individual.

This same approach can be utilized regardless of the material being reviewed or relearned. It is probably not realistic for individuals to always plan learning experiences based solely on their learning style preferences; however, consistent use of a preferred learning style will tend to maximize a candidate's efficiency during his/her preparation for the Physical Therapist Examination.

The knowledge acquired about your learning environment preferences can assist you in creating a productive study atmosphere when working alone or with others. It also can assist you in selecting an appropriate study partner and/or indicate whether you are a good candidate for group learning.

The knowledge acquired about thinking mode preferences will apply directly to the questions on the Physical Therapist Examination. Since the examination emphasizes clinically oriented material, it requires integrated thinking. Candidates must not only know cognitive information, but they must also demonstrate performance proficiency. Suggestions for an effective information gathering system to achieve integration will be presented in Unit Five.

If you determined you were left-brain dominant on the thinking mode exercise, you probably will be more comfortable answering questions that demonstrate more of a left-brain bias. Conversely, if you are right-brain dominant, you probably will be more comfortable answering questions that demonstrate more of a right-brain bias. Examination questions, although usually requiring integrated thinking, still may have a left or right-brain bias. By being familiar with the characteristics of both left and right-brain questions, candidates can develop an increased awareness of their own learning style and develop particular learning activities directed toward their non-dominant thinking mode.

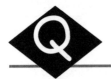

Sample Questions

The following section provides three sample questions. As you read each of the questions, take note of those which are easy for you and those which are more of a challenge, and see if you can determine why. A brief analysis of each question is presented, along with an answer key at the conclusion of the exercise.

Each of the answer keys throughout the text lists the best answer to each question and identifies a resource which supports the stated answer. In the vast majority of cases a page number is also provided to direct candidates to the appropriate subject matter. The complete reference for each of the resources is located in the bibliography.

Sample Question One:
A physical therapist examines a patient that has burns over her anterior right arm, the anterior portion of the thorax, and the genital region. Based on the "rule of nines", what percentage of the patient's body is affected?

1. 19.0%
2. 22.5%
3. 23.5%
4. 28.0%

Analysis: This question will tend to favor left-brain dominant candidates. The question requires candidates to recall detailed information, specifically the percentage of the total body surface allocated to the nine various anatomical segments.

Sample Question Two:

A physical therapist observes a patient ambulating in the physical therapy gym. The therapist notes that the patient's pelvis drops on the right during left stance phase. In an attempt to compensate, the patient laterally bends his trunk over the stance leg. This type of gait deviation can be caused by weakness of the:

1. gluteus maximus
2. gluteus medius
3. iliopsoas
4. tensor fasciae latae

Analysis: This question will tend to favor right-brain dominant candidates. The question requires candidates to identify the relationship between a specific muscle function and a resultant gait deviation.

Sample Question Three:

A physical therapist is treating a six-month-old infant with spina bifida. The infant suddenly begins to act strangely during the treatment session. A primary survey reveals the infant is not breathing, but does have a pulse. The most immediate response would be to:

1. begin chest compressions
2. begin mouth to mouth breathing
3. begin mouth to nose breathing
4. begin mouth to mouth and nose breathing

Analysis: This question is more representative of the integrated type that will make up the majority of the Physical Therapist Examination. This specific question requires candidates not only to be familiar with the sequential steps of cardiopulmonary resuscitation, but also to recognize the relationship among a number of other factors including when a patient has a pulse and is not breathing. The candidate is further required to identify the most immediate response.

Answer Key

1. Answer: 3   Resource: O'Sullivan (p. 852)
   The percentage of the total body surface burned in an adult can be calculated using the rule of nines: anterior right arm 4.5%, anterior portion of the thorax 18%, genital region 1%. Total = 23.5%

2. Answer: 2   Resource: Magee (p. 866)
   The gluteus medius muscle is a hip abductor. Weakness of the abductor can result in a Trendelenburg gait.

3. Answer: 4   Resource: American Heart Association
                                                    (p. 148)
   Mouth to mouth and nose breathing is utilized on an infant (less than one year).

As you progress through the sample questions in this text, it should become apparent that to be successful on the examination, a candidate will have to demonstrate both left and right-brain proficiency. It is therefore advisable for a candidate's study plan to incorporate activities which utilize both left-brain and right-brain thinking modes.

We will continue to expand on many of the topics we have introduced throughout the text. Included in the following unit will be general and specific study guidelines and specific learning style recommendations.

Study Plan

The simple thought of preparing for a comprehensive examination such as the Physical Therapist Examination can be overwhelming. Many candidates ask themselves how it is possible to prepare adequately for an examination that encompasses more than two years of professional coursework.

One of the largest advantages of taking an examination such as the Physical Therapist Examination is that it does not require candidates to demonstrate mastery of new material. On the surface this may not seem like a significant advantage, but since candidates are, in effect, only reviewing or relearning previously presented information, their level of attainment should be significantly greater.

Many candidates fail to utilize this advantage. Candidates who attempt to learn large quantities of new information, instead of focusing on understanding and applying basic concepts, often do themselves a tremendous disservice. It is true that there undoubtedly will be questions that contain information that was not part of a selected curriculum, but to attempt to study this new information in any significant detail would be a large mistake for most candidates. Instead, candidates should focus on reviewing or relearning basic concepts that are an integral component of all accredited physical therapy programs. It is this type of information that will make up the vast majority of the examination. Individuals who take this common sense approach optimize their chances of success on this important examination.

Developing a Plan

Developing a study plan allows candidates to take control of their preparation. Candidates should begin by compiling a list of all the necessary topics that must be reviewed prior to the examination. The topics should be assembled in a sequence that will allow for a smooth transition between topics. Candidates should make an estimate of the time needed to review each topic and compile a list of available resources.

The Reporter's Formula

Throughout history, individuals have been sent out to gather information about ideas, events, processes, and people. To assist these individuals, a specific formula was developed. This formula was termed "the reporter's formula."

The reporter's formula contains the following seven question words: Who, What, Which, When, Where, How, and Why. This time tested technique of information gathering can be utilized by candidates preparing for the Physical Therapist Examination in a number of different ways:

1. Incorporate the formula into a study plan for each content category
2. Utilize the formula as an outline for study sessions
3. Generate potential examination questions using the formula

The formula also can be used to categorize actual examination questions. This specific technique will be explored in detail in Unit Five.

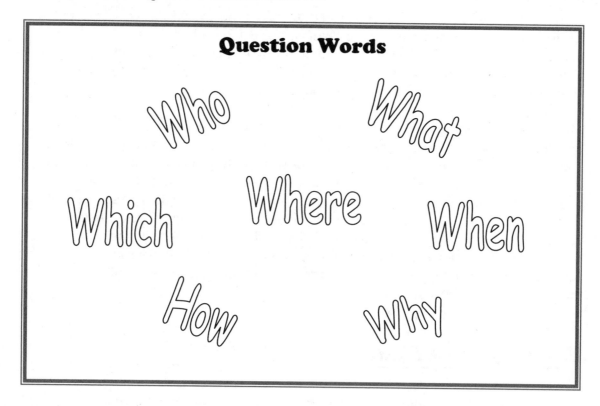

Goals

Before beginning to study, develop specific goals for each study session. Ideally, these goals should be established on a weekly basis. Establishing goals will ensure that candidates cover the desired material and will serve as a mechanism to keep them on schedule with their study plan. Candidates should be realistic with the goals they establish and should not attempt to cover more material than is possible in a particular study session.

Reviewing

Reviewing is defined operationally as looking over or studying previously learned information. Reviewing can play an important role in a candidate's preparation for the Physical Therapist Examination. It is recommended that students review classnotes for their practice oriented professional coursework. Practice oriented professional coursework typically includes, but is not limited to, study of the musculoskeletal, neuromuscular, cardiopulmonary, and integumentary systems. In addition, candidates usually have coursework in patient care skills, physical agents, administration, ethics, research, and education. Each of these topics are important components of the content outline for the Physical Therapist Examination.

Classnotes may seem voluminous to candidates, but they can be reviewed fairly quickly. Special attention must be taken not to become bogged down in one specific area for any significant amount of time. General concepts that are understood should be scanned quickly, while other concepts that are more difficult for a candidate should be read carefully. Concepts that remain unclear after being reviewed should be written down for future study sessions.

Other foundational coursework encountered earlier in the professional curriculum can be consulted as needed during various study sessions. This type of coursework often includes, but is not limited to Anatomy and Physiology, Neuroanatomy, Exercise Physiology, and Kinesiology. It is important to limit the amount of time spent reviewing this type of foundational coursework. Candidates often can make better use of their allotted time by reviewing coursework encountered later in the curriculum that may be more practice oriented. By reviewing practice oriented information, candidates not only keep their studying consistent with the format of the examination, but at the same time indirectly review much of the information presented in the foundational coursework.

Relearning

Relearning is defined operationally as reacquiring knowledge or comprehension which was known previously. Relearning is often a necessary component of a comprehensive study plan. In physical therapy academic programs, candidates constantly are learning new information on a variety of topics. Although students typically exhibit mastery of selected material during a scheduled examination, they do not always retain the information for later use. Failure to retain information that was learned previously is the primary rationale for relearning.

Relearning can take place in a variety of ways. Often times, simply reviewing information is enough for candidates to relearn the material; however, in some cases, a more indepth approach is necessary. This approach may include using textbooks, class handouts, and interacting with classmates or professors. It is imperative that candidates relearn material which may be an integral component of the examination. It must be stressed, however, that to focus on memorizing minuscule facts or inordinate details would be, at best, poor utilization of available study time.

Journal

It is recommended that candidates keep a daily journal of their studying. This journal should include a variety of information:

1. Topics/concepts that were reviewed successfully
2. Topics/concepts requiring additional review or relearning
3. List of goals for each study session
4. Progress towards meeting established goals
5. Resources utilized during the study session
6. Plan for the subsequent study session

As candidates begin to complete sample examinations, the journal will allow them to document specific information on their performance. This should include the percentage of questions answered correctly and the amount of time necessary to complete a selected examination. Candidates should survey questions that were answered incorrectly and attempt to determine if there are any general patterns. For example, if a candidate consistently has difficulty answering questions related to a specific topic area or questions that were constructed in a similar manner, these deficits should be recorded. Once identified, appropriate remedial strategies can be developed.

General Recommendations

To this point, candidates have learned a variety of strategies to utilize when developing a study plan for the Physical Therapist Examination. There are, however, a variety of other variables that can influence the quality of a study session. This text will describe many of these variables.

Environment

To construct an optimal learning environment, candidates should attempt to incorporate their individual learning preferences into each study session. Return to Unit Three to reexamine the preferences best suited for your specific concentration and learning needs.

Supplies

Gather the necessary supplies to assist you in studying. Begin the study session with all of the necessary supplies to complete the entire session. Unnecessary breaks to gather additional resources will only serve to prolong or limit the effectiveness of your study session.

Timing

We all function more effectively at specific times of the day. Ideally, study sessions should take place when the mind is alert and attentive. Select a time during the day when you feel you are at your optimal level of functioning. Avoid studying when you are physically tired. Activities such as eating or heavy exercise can lead to decreased attentiveness, and as a result, decrease the effectiveness of your study session. Make sure your emotional state is conducive to learning. If you have had a particularly bad day, avoid studying. Study sessions tend to be unproductive when a candidate is less than 100 percent emotionally.

Frequency and Duration

Studying for short intervals of time has proven to be a more effective learning strategy than studying for long intervals. Specific parameters for frequency and duration are not provided, since they can vary considerably for different learning styles and purposes.

Partnership and Group Recommendations

Many candidates can significantly enhance their preparation for the Physical Therapist Examination by participating in a study partnership or group. This type of collaboration can offer candidates several distinct benefits:

- Candidates can learn from the information presented by others and as a result reduce their individual study time.

- Candidates can receive assistance from others when remediation is necessary.

- Candidates can assess and modify their individual study plan based on the perceptions and knowledge of others.

Although these arrangements have the potential to be a valuable component of a comprehensive study plan, they need to be structured in a fashion that will allow candidates to be productive. Failure to have adequate structure can result in a study session degenerating into a purely social event. To avoid this potential pitfall, we recommend the following guidelines for all partnerships or groups:

1. Set rules of behavior and a method for staying on task.

2. Set the length and frequency of study sessions, keeping in mind your long-range plan.

3. Set goals that indicate the amount of material to be covered in a specified time period.

4. Establish time during scheduled study sessions to address individual learning needs.

5. Discuss and agree on an agenda for each scheduled study session.

6. Decide on the structure of each study session:

Hierarchical: Someone acts as "teacher" for each session
Participative: Each member acts as facilitator for an area of study
Debate: Exchange of ideas after independent study

7. Attempt to institute a firm schedule for study sessions and emphasize the importance of attendance at each session.

8. Decide on the learning tools the partnership/group will use during each study session.

Candidates should take advantage of available resources, but at the same time recognize there are limits to this type of collaborative approach. It is illegal and unethical to solicit questions from candidates who have taken the examination or to recall and share questions with other candidates after taking the examination. The Federation of State Boards of Physical Therapy will actively prosecute individuals who are engaged in such activities.

Learning Style

The following section offers candidates specific recommendations based on their individual input/processing preferences. Candidates should attempt to utilize this information when participating in a study partnership or group.

Active/Active

Format:
Study sessions should consist of 60-90 minutes of interactive study. The sessions should be designed based on the categories contained within the content outline. Candidates should divide the content outline into smaller, more manageable components.

Many active learners will find it helpful to develop three specific concepts, ideas, or processes to work on for each scheduled study session. After the study session is completed, candidates should make sure they have achieved each established goal. Ample time should be allotted at the end of the study session for a brief review.

Active/Active learners often prefer to divide the workload for the next session. These tasks typically are done independently and usually involve reviewing selected material that will be discussed as part of the next session. This same routine can be repeated with each study session until the actual examination.

Group Composition:
Group members should include learners who are active for input, or processing, or both. There should be a representative sample of left-brain (facts, details) and right-brain (big picture, relationships) dominant candidates.

Frequency:
Since multisensory stimulation is more difficult to achieve alone, it is recommended that study sessions take place as frequently as possible. Daily study sessions would not be considered excessive.

Concerns:
Effective time management is critical, because it can take considerably longer to achieve multisensory stimulation.

Learning Tools:
Color-coding may help in stimulating the visual channel. Discussions, simulations, hands-on practice, and role playing are viable learning activities.

- **Left-brain:** lists, outlines, flow charts
- **Right-brain:** charts, graphs, mind maps

Tips:
Position yourself so that you can observe body language during the study session. Videotapes of sessions may be useful to play back during individual study time to help recreate the study session.

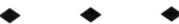

Active/Passive

Format:
Study sessions should be scheduled for a maximum of two hours. The sessions should be designed based on the categories contained within the content outline. Candidates should divide the content outline into smaller, more manageable components.

Many active learners will find it helpful to develop three specific concepts, ideas or processes to work on for each scheduled study session. After the study session is completed, candidates should make sure they have achieved each established goal.

Ample time should be allotted at the end of the study session for a brief review, and specific tasks should be delegated for the following study session. These tasks typically are done independently and usually involve reviewing selected material that will be discussed as part of the next study session. This same routine can be repeated with each study session until the actual examination.

Although most Active/Passive learners prefer to review information themselves, we recommend that they use a participative format for group work. In this format, each member assumes responsibility for an area of study. Group activity will limit the detailed studying these learners prefer, and provide them with a more comprehensive understanding of the presented material.

Group Composition:
Group members should include learners who are active for input, or processing, or both. There should be a representative sample of left-brain (facts, details) and right-brain (big picture, relationships) dominant candidates.

Frequency:
Two to three times per week is recommended. Candidates may have a desire to reduce the number of sessions; however, they are best served by frequent meetings.

Concerns:
Time management is necessary to maintain concentration and allow for a smooth progression through the content outline.

Learning Tools:
Color-coding may help in stimulating the visual channel. Discussions, simulations, hands-on practice, role playing, and blackboard "teaching" are viable examples.

- **Left-brain:** lists, outlines, flow charts
- **Right-brain:** charts, graphs, mind maps

Tips:
Position yourself so that you can observe body language during the study session. Videotapes of sessions may be useful to play back during individual study time to help recreate the study session.

Passive/Active

Format:
Since the majority of studying will take place independently, study sessions should function as an opportunity for candidates to assess their current study plan and benefit from the knowledge of others.

Study sessions should range from two to three hours in length and should focus on large pieces of material. An example of this would be a session at the conclusion of a major section of the content outline.

Group Composition:
Group members should include learners who prefer to study alone and then gather to discuss specific information. Both left and right-brain dominant candidates should be included in the group.

Frequency:
Approximately once per week is recommended. This schedule will allow candidates to cover the necessary material within the established time parameters.

Concerns:
Since the majority of studying has been completed before the review sessions, candidates need to be very careful to include both concepts and applications in their study plan.

Learning Tools:
Blackboard presentations, briefings, debate, occasional simulations.

- **Left-brain:** outlines, lists, flow charts
- **Right-brain:** charts, graphs, mind maps

Tips:
Candidates may have little patience with partners or group members who come to sessions unprepared.

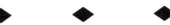

Passive/Passive

Format:
Since the majority of studying will take place independently, study sessions should function as an opportunity for candidates to assess their current study plan and benefit from the knowledge of others.

Study sessions should range from two to three hours in length and should focus on large pieces of material. An example of this would be a session at the conclusion of a major section of the content outline. Since candidates' focus in this category is not on application of material, they should make sure that this area is addressed at each study session.

Group Composition:
Group members should include individuals who prefer to study alone initially. The group should also include members who are application driven.

Frequency:
Approximately once per week is recommended. This schedule will allow candidates to cover the necessary material within the established time parameters.

Concerns:
Time management is necessary to maintain concentration and limit the role of stress.

Learning Tools:
Lectures, blackboard presentations, briefings, observation of simulations, handouts, texts, notes.

- **Left-brain:** outlines, lists, flow charts
- **Right-brain:** charts, graphs, mind maps

Tips:
Passive/Passive learners may become very uncomfortable physically engaging in learning activities before having a chance to review and observe.

Multiple Choice Examinations

Do you believe that Jason Giambi was hitting 450 foot homeruns as a little leaguer or that Serena Williams was consistently hitting blistering passing shots in the second grade? Your answer to these questions is likely to be no. Since history tells us these individuals later accomplished the aforementioned feats, the question becomes, what allowed these individuals to progress to such lofty heights?

The answer probably can best be described in a single word, "practice." Surely individuals like Jason Giambi and Serena Williams were blessed with certain athletic and physical traits which provided them with the opportunity to become successful, but it was their dedication, desire, and determination that allowed them to evolve into superstars in their respective fields.

In physical therapy, there are an abundance of skills that must be learned by the entry level practitioner. Mastery of these skills often requires physical therapists to demonstrate the same type of dedication, desire, and determination exhibited by Jason Giambi and Serena Williams.

Test taking skills are specific skills which allow individuals to utilize the characteristics and format of a selected examination in order to maximize their performance. These skills can be valuable when taking an examination such as the Physical Therapist Examination. Despite the importance of this topic, very little, if any, academic time is set aside to address test taking skills. The good news is that test taking skills can be learned and that through dedication, desire, and determination, these skills can serve to improve your performance on this important examination.

Since the Physical Therapist Examination utilizes a multiple choice format, further discussion of test taking skills will be solely concerned with this particular format. Test taking skills can allow candidates to increase their ability to recognize cues within the multiple choice questions. These cues can be utilized to provide valuable information toward identifying the correct response. It has been documented in the literature that recognition of selected cues can lead to improved examination performance.

Individuals who are able to recognize such cues are said to be "test wise." Perhaps this explains, in part, why many students who have prepared adequately for a selected examination often perform poorly. Test taking skills are acquired skills that develop with practice. This unit will present candidates with valuable information on multiple choice examinations and a variety of test taking skills. The unit will also provide candidates with an opportunity to apply the described test taking skills on selected sample examination questions.

Multiple Choice Questions

The Physical Therapist Examination is a 225 question multiple choice examination that consists of 200 scored items and 25 pretest items. The objective examination consists of multiple choice questions with four potentially correct answers to each question. Candidates are instructed to select the "best answer" to complete each question.

Before we begin to explore selected test taking strategies, we need to identify the various components of a multiple choice question. Multiple choice questions can be dissected into specific identifiable components:

Item: An item refers to an individual multiple choice question and the corresponding potential answers.

Stem: The stem refers to the statement that asks the question.

Options: Options refer to the potential answers to the question asked. One option in each item will be the "best answer," while the others are distracters.

Item:
The Physical Therapist Examination contains 200 scored items and 25 pretest items. Each item consists of a stem and four options. Items may vary considerably in content and length, but should utilize a consistent format.

Stem:
The stem can take on a variety of forms. Typically, the stem conveys to the reader the necessary information needed to respond correctly to the question. In addition to the necessary information, many times extraneous information is included in the stem. This information, when not recognized by the candidate as unnecessary, often can act as a significant distracter.

The stem commonly can take on the form of a complete sentence, an incomplete sentence, or a fill-in-the-blank. The stem can be expressed in a positive or negative form. A positive form would require a candidate to identify correct information, while a negative form would require a candidate to identify incorrect information. It is important to scrutinize each stem, since a single key word such as "not" or "except" can turn a positive stem into a negative stem. Failure to identify this can lead to the identification of an incorrect answer.

Options:

Options can take on a variety of forms, including a single word, a group of words, an incomplete sentence, a complete sentence, or a group of sentences. The method for analyzing each option does not change, regardless of form.

Question Categorization System

Let's take a few moments to review what we already have learned about the Physical Therapist Examination. We know that the examination consists of 225 multiple choice questions, each with four possible options. We also know that each question will be representative of one of the four content areas identified in the content outline.

As we introduced in Unit Four, the reporter's formula can be a valuable tool to assist candidates with their preparation for the examination. The reporter's formula utilizes seven specific question words: Who, What, Which, Where, When, How, and Why. By relating each of the question words to the material in the content outline, candidates can effectively review the majority of the information that will be encountered on the Physical Therapist Examination. By reviewing the information in this manner, candidates gather and store the information in an organized and efficient fashion.

This system can also be utilized to a candidate's advantage when analyzing a multiple choice question. As candidates analyze specific examination questions, they should attempt to categorize each question using the same seven question words. By identifying the correct question word for each of the multiple choice questions, candidates are, in effect, telling the brain where to access the desired information. Since a candidate's study plan was designed in a similar fashion, this process will improve the rate and fluidity of information retrieval. On a timed examination such as the Physical Therapist Examination, this can be a significant advantage.

It is important for candidates to remember that the purpose of the question categorization system is to assist candidates in understanding the intended meaning of each question. By understanding exactly what each question is asking, candidates can avoid making careless mistakes and improve their examination performance.

Four Levels of Learning & Related Question Types

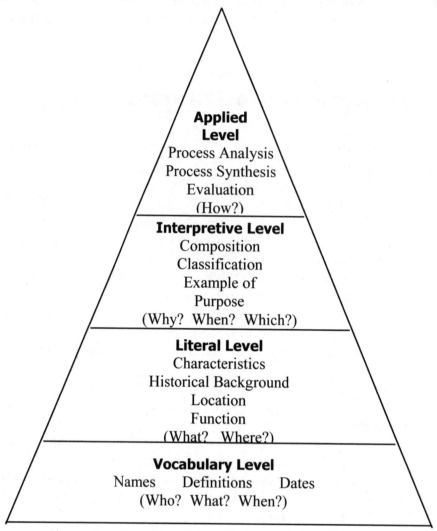

Figure adapted by and reprinted with the permission of Linda Lyon.

Of course, we have oversimplified the process, but in your mind you should begin to see how this information can be applied effectively to the Physical Therapist Examination.

In an attempt to allow candidates to accurately classify examination items, we have divided the seven question words into five separate categories. Selected sample examination questions will be offered to illustrate the use of each category.

Each item in this section will deal with vital signs. Remember, to be classified into a specific category, the exact question word associated with the category does not have to be utilized; rather, think in terms of the problem solving process or the information required to answer the question.

Exercise One

The following exercise contains eleven sample questions for candidates to answer. An answer key is located at the conclusion of the exercise.

Who

This category contains information concerning specific individuals who have made various contributions to the field of physical therapy. It also could include information related to a specific discipline or the responsibilities associated with the discipline.

Sample Question One:

A physical therapist works on an interdisciplinary team in an acute care hospital. One of the patients scheduled to be treated has had severe fluctuations in her blood pressure throughout the night and has been monitored by the nursing staff. Which interdisciplinary team member would be the most appropriate to determine the patient's ability to complete her scheduled rehabilitative session?

1. physical therapist
2. occupational therapist
3. nurse
4. physician

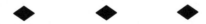

What/Which

This category contains information associated with facts and details. Learning this information typically requires memorization.

What/Which information can be divided into five separate categories:

- Definition
- Characteristics
- Classification
- Composition
- Example

Definition: *meanings of words, terms or procedures*

Sample Question Two:
A physical therapist reviews the medical record of a patient scheduled to be examined in physical therapy. An entry in the medical record indicates the patient has tachycardia. Which description most accurately defines tachycardia?

1. an abnormally fast heart rate
2. an abnormally slow heart rate
3. shortness of breath
4. labored or difficult breathing

Characteristics: *distinguishing traits, qualities, or properties*

Sample Question Three:
A physical therapist records the vital signs of a 42-year-old female at rest. The patient was referred to physical therapy after sustaining a trimalleolar fracture. Which of the following values would not be considered within normal limits?

1. pulse: 82 beats per minute
2. blood pressure: 122/85 mm Hg
3. respiration rate: 20 respirations per minute
4. body temperature: 97.8 °F

Classification: *arranging in, or assigning to, various groups, classes or categories*

Sample Question Four:
A physical therapist measures the blood pressure of a 68-year-old male. The therapist determines the patient's blood pressure is 124/84 mm Hg. This value is best classified as:

1. mild hypotension
2. mild hypertension
3. moderate hypertension
4. within normal limits

Composition: *identifying individual elements or arrangements*

Sample Question Five:
A physical therapist attempts to calculate a patient's age predicted maximum heart rate. Which of the following is utilized as a component of the age predicted maximum heart rate formula?

1. 180
2. 200
3. 220
4. 240

Example: *a representative sample*

Sample Question Six:
A physical therapist determines that a patient's blood pressure is elevated when comparing the value obtained during a recent measurement to the patient's normal resting value. Which of the following would tend to increase resting blood pressure?

1. medication
2. anxiety
3. loss of blood
4. decreased cardiac output

Where

Information in this category usually refers to a location.

Sample Question Seven:
A physical therapist assesses a patient's pulse. In order to accurately assess the patient's apical pulse, the therapist should position the stethoscope:

1. on the chest wall over the apex of the heart
2. over the femoral artery
3. over the carotid artery
4. over the posterior tibial artery

As you can see by answering the Who, What, Which, and Where questions for each of the content areas, there will be very little information that will be omitted from your review. However, you also should recognize that the majority of the material contained within these question words has dealt with fact based information and has not emphasized clinical application. The next series of categories will be more prevalent on the Physical Therapist Examination. They will deal almost exclusively with clinical application.

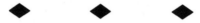

How/When

Information in this category involves processes; specifically how to perform tasks step by step and how to analyze what has been done. In some cases, the information follows a sequential timeline (whole-to-part) and sometimes it necessitates drawing together diverse information (part-to-whole) and forming a conclusion.

How/When information can be divided into two categories:

- Process Analysis
- Process Synthesis

Process Analysis: *step by step sequencing of information or actions*

Sample Question Eight:

A patient sitting in a chair in the physical therapy waiting room suddenly falls to the floor and appears to be unconscious. The physical therapist determines that the patient is not breathing and administers two rescue breaths. The therapist then checks the patient's carotid pulse. If the therapist is able to detect a pulse, he/she should next:

1. begin external chest compressions
2. continue rescue breathing
3. readjust the head tilt and attempt to ventilate
4. determine the pulse rate for 60 seconds

Process Synthesis: *merging of information into "the big picture" and making an informed "action plan"*

Sample Question Nine:

A patient with tetraplegia is two weeks status post cervical spinal fusion. After transferring the patient from the bed to a wheelchair, the patient complains of a severe headache. Upon examination, the patient is found to be diaphoretic and flushed. The patient's blood pressure is recorded as 210/130 mm Hg. These signs and symptoms are most indicative of:

1. autonomic dysreflexia
2. urinary tract infection
3. orthostatic hypotension
4. pulmonary embolus

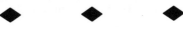

Why

This category typically requires a more advanced level of knowledge than many of the other categories. To answer a Why question successfully, it may be necessary to answer simultaneously What, Which, Where, and/or How information.

Why information can be divided into two categories:

- Cause and Effect
- Function/Use Concepts

Cause and Effect: *relationship between an outcome or state of being and the causative factors*

Sample Question Ten:

A physical therapist attempts to assess the blood pressure of a grossly obese patient. If the bladder of the blood pressure cuff used is too narrow in relation to the circumference of the patient's arm, which of the following would best describe the resultant effect on the patient's measured blood pressure?

1. the value will be erroneously low
2. the value will be erroneously high
3. the value will be reflective of the patient's actual blood pressure
4. the value will not be reflective of the patient's actual blood pressure

Function/Use Concepts: explanation or rationale for a selected action

Sample Question Eleven:

A physical therapist establishes a baseline measurement of a patient's vital signs prior to beginning a phase II cardiac rehabilitation program. The primary purpose of conducting the baseline measurement is to:

1. determine the therapeutic measures most appropriate for the patient's rehabilitation program
2. demonstrate objective progress in the patient's rehabilitation program
3. protect the therapist from unnecessary litigation
4. identify significant changes in the values as a result of exercise or other factors

It is possible that many of the examination questions will fall into more than one of the question categories.

Answer Key

1. Answer: 4   Resource: Guide for Professional
                                                         Conduct
   Severe fluctuations in blood pressure can be indicative of a serious medical condition.   The physician is the appropriate professional to assess the patient's changing medical status.

2. Answer: 1   Resource: Minor (p. 39)
   Tachycardia is an abnormally fast heart rate, greater than 100 beats per minute.

3. Answer: 3   Resource: Pierson (p. 59)
   Normal respiration rate in an adult is 12-18 breaths per minute.

4. Answer: 4   Resource: Minor (p. 42)
   124/84 mm Hg is within the accepted blood pressure range for adults.

5. Answer: 3   Resource: Kisner (p. 167)
   Age predicted maximum heart rate is defined as 220 minus age.

6. Answer: 2   Resource: Pierson (p. 59)
   Blood pressure will increase with anxiety and other significant changes in emotional status. Medication may increase or decrease resting blood pressure.

7. Answer: 1　　　　　　　　Resource: Pierson (p. 47)
Auscultation over the apex of the heart using a stethoscope can be used to assess the apical pulse.

8. Answer: 2　　　　　　　　Resource: American Heart Association (p. 75)
Rescue breathing is indicated for a patient that is not breathing, however does have a detectable pulse.

9. Answer: 1　　　　　　　　Resource: Pierson (p. 335)
Autonomic dysreflexia is an exaggerated reflex of the autonomic nervous system. It often occurs in individuals with recent spinal cord injuries and is characterized by severe hypertension, headache, and sweating.

10. Answer: 2　　　　　　　　Resource: Pierson (p. 56)
A narrow blood pressure cuff will cause the measured value to be high. The width of the bladder should be 40% of the circumference of the midpoint of the limb.

11. Answer: 4　　　　　　　　Resource: Brannon (p. 250)
Significant changes in vital signs can only be determined when compared to baseline values. This is a fundamental component of all cardiac rehabilitation programs.

Task Approach

On the Physical Therapist Examination there are 225 items that candidates must answer within a four and one half hour time period. Due to the length of the examination and the time constraints associated with it, candidates need to approach the examination in a systematic and organized fashion. Loss of control during the examination will yield poor results that are not reflective of a candidate's actual knowledge. We will introduce a four phase process as an example of an approach that can be used effectively when answering examination questions in a review text or, with slight modification, on a computer based test.

Phase I
Carefully read the stem of the first item. Underline key words or groups of words that offer valuable information. Circle command words that indicate the desired action. If after reading the stem, you are able to generate an answer to the item, make a mental note or write the hypothesized answer on scratch paper.

Candidates should then begin to examine each option one at a time. It is important to read the entire option, since one word often can make a potentially correct answer incorrect. If the generated answer is consistent with one of the available options, the candidate should give the option strong consideration; however since more than one option can be correct it is imperative to analyze each presented option. If candidates are not able to generate a response, regardless of the reason, they should place an asterisk next to the item number and move to the next item.

Since computer based testing does not allow candidates to mark desired words or phrases, they need to make use of several less direct indicators. These indicators usually take the form of a mental note or a brief written message.

Phase II

Once candidates have completed all of the questions to which they can generate an answer, they should progress to a true/false format. This format allows candidates to have only one potential option in front of them at a time, therefore significantly limiting the distracters.

Candidates should begin by uncovering one of the available options and saying to themselves, "Is it true that ...?" Be sure to substitute the key terms and command words from the stem. Place a "T" or "F" next to the selected option and move to the next option. Continue this pattern until all of the available options have been analyzed. If, after applying this technique, an answer becomes apparent, the candidate should select the answer. If the answer is not apparent, the candidate should move to the next question.

Phase III

By the time a candidate progresses to this phase, the vast majority of the questions on the examination should have been answered. Candidates should return to the beginning of the examination and revisit each remaining question with an asterisk. Candidates again should attempt to generate a response to each of the questions. Likewise, candidates should attempt to analyze unanswered questions by revisiting the true/false format.

Phase IV

At this point there should be very few remaining unanswered questions. Candidates now must utilize deductive reasoning strategies to answer the remaining questions. Deductive reasoning strategies allow candidates to secure points beyond those acquired through direct knowledge of subject matter. Although deductive reasoning strategies are not meant to be used in place of academic knowledge, they have proven to be an effective strategy to improve examination performance.

Deductive reasoning strategies often allow candidates to eliminate one or more of the potential answers. Elimination of any option significantly increases the probability of identifying the correct answer. On the Physical Therapist Examination, eliminating one option increases the chance of selecting a correct answer from 25% to 33%. Eliminating two options increases the chance of selecting a correct answer to 50%. On the surface this may not seem terribly significant, however on a 200 question test such as the Physical Therapist Examination this can be the difference between a passing and a failing score. Selected deductive reasoning strategies that can be used effectively on the Physical Therapist Examination are presented.

- **Absurd Options:** Many times a multiple choice item will include an option that is not consistent with what the stem is asking or with the other options. In many cases, this option can be eliminated. Rapid elimination of specific options will allow candidates to spend additional time analyzing other more viable options.

- **Similar Options:** When two or more options have a similar meaning or express the same fact, they often imply each other's incorrectness. Since candidates are instructed to select the best answer, it would be extremely unlikely that one of two options that are so close in resemblance would be the correct answer. For this reason, candidates can often eliminate both options.

- **Obtainable Information:** There is a great deal of factual material that candidates must sift through when taking the Physical Therapist Examination. In some instances, the material can provide candidates with valuable information that can assist them in answering other examination questions.

- **Errors in Test Construction:** Since many different individuals are involved in developing the Physical Therapist Examination, it is difficult to make generalizations about examination construction. Candidates should attempt to answer each question exactly as it is written and avoid the temptation to speculate on the intention of the author.

- **Degree of Qualification:** Particularly in the sciences, there seem to be many exceptions to general rules. Therefore, specific determiners such as "always" or "never" often over qualify an option.

- **Position of the Correct Answer:** Research has demonstrated the tendency for the correct answer in a sequence of alternatives to be at the center of the response distribution. On the Physical Therapist Examination, the center of the response distribution would correlate to answers 2 and 3.

It is important to remember that deductive reasoning strategies should not be used as a substitute for academic knowledge. Deductive reasoning strategies, when applied indiscriminately or as a substitute for academic knowledge, lead to poor results. Deductive reasoning strategies should be applied only when candidates are unable to identify the correct response using academic knowledge. In these instances, deductive reasoning strategies can be used in combination with academic knowledge to increase the probability of selecting the best answer to a specific examination item.

If after progressing through the four phase process, a candidate still is unable to make an informed decision, he/she should simply attempt to guess at the correct answer. Since there is no penalty associated with guessing on the Physical Therapist Examination, it is in a candidate's best interest to answer each question.

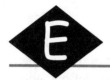

Exercise Two

In this exercise, three sample questions are presented. Candidates should attempt to identify the best answer to each question by utilizing the four phase process. Candidates should also attempt to identify the question type and the specific content area.

The following tables list the possible responses in each category:

Question Category	Content Outline
Who	Examination
What/Which	Evaluation, Diagnosis, Prognosis, and Outcomes
Where	Intervention
How/When	Standards of Care
Why	

An analysis section immediately follows each of the three sample questions. The analysis section begins by showing the sample question with key terms underlined and command words in bold type. A brief narrative follows, which describes how the four phase process can be applied to the sample question.

An answer key located at the conclusion of the exercise indicates the best answer, question type, and content category for each of the sample questions.

Sample Question One:

A physical therapist instructs a patient with a Foley catheter in ambulation activities. During ambulation the therapist should position the collection bag:

1. above the level of the patient's bladder
2. below the level of the patient's bladder
3. above the level of the patient's heart
4. below the level of the patient's heart

Analysis:

A physical therapist instructs a patient with a <u>Foley catheter in ambulation activities</u>. During ambulation the therapist should **position** <u>the collection bag</u>:

1. above the level of the patient's bladder
2. below the level of the patient's bladder
3. above the level of the patient's heart
4. below the level of the patient's heart

After reading the stem and identifying the pertinent information a candidate should attempt to generate an answer. The candidate then should begin to reveal each of the available options. If a generated answer is consistent with one of the available options, there is a high probability that the answer is correct.

If a candidate was not able to generate an answer, he/she should progress to a true/false format. The candidate will begin this process by creating a true/false statement for each of the available options. The true/false statement for option "1" would be as follows:

Is it true that during ambulation the therapist should position the collection bag above the level of the patient's bladder?

The candidate should answer each question by placing a "T" or "F" next to the corresponding option. He/she should then progress through all of the remaining options in the same manner. Remember, it is possible to have more than one option which satisfactorily answers the question. It is then the candidate's responsibility to select the best answer from the viable options.

Sample Question Two:

A group of physical therapists attempts to determine the relationship between two variables on an examination form. Which of the following correlation coefficients would indicate the strongest relationship?

1. +.86
2. +.45
3. -.34
4. -.89

Analysis:

A group of physical therapists attempts to determine <u>the relationship between two variables</u> on an examination form. Which of the following <u>correlation coefficients</u> would indicate the **strongest relationship**?

1. +.86
2. +.45
3. -.34
4. -.89

After reading the stem and identifying the pertinent information, a candidate should recognize that it is virtually impossible to generate an answer prior to viewing the available options. A candidate should, however, begin to think about correlation coefficients and determining the strength of the relationship between variables.

The candidate should then begin to expose each of the available options. Since, in this specific example, all of the options are numerical, it will not be particularly helpful to apply a true/false format. Instead, a candidate should examine the possible options and attempt to identify the correct response.

Although the four phase process does not directly supply a candidate with the correct response, by carefully reading the stem, a candidate can avoid an unnecessary mistake. In this item, the stem asks the candidate to identify the correlation coefficient that indicates the strongest relationship between the two variables. If a candidate does not read the question carefully, he/she may make an assumption that the stem is asking for the strongest positive relationship and subsequently answer the question incorrectly.

It is important that a candidate answer each item based only on the given information. By making even small assumptions or by not reading each item carefully, a candidate can make careless mistakes.

Sample Question Three:

A physical therapist completes an isokinetic examination on an 18-year-old male rehabilitating from a medial meniscectomy. The therapist notes that the patient generates 140 ft/lbs of force using the uninvolved quadriceps at 60 degrees per second. Assuming a normal ratio of hamstrings to quadriceps strength, which of the following would be an acceptable hamstrings value at 60 degrees per second?

1. 64 ft/lbs
2. 84 ft/lbs
3. 114 ft/lbs
4. 116 ft/lbs

Analysis:

A physical therapist completes an isokinetic examination on an 18-year-old male rehabilitating from a medial meniscectomy. The therapist notes that the patient generates 140 ft/lbs of force using the uninvolved quadriceps at 60 degrees per second. Assuming a normal ratio of hamstrings to quadriceps strength, which of the following would be **an acceptable hamstrings value** at 60 degrees per second?

1. 64 ft/lbs
2. 84 ft/lbs
3. 114 ft/lbs
4. 116 ft/lbs

For the purpose of discussion, let's assume a candidate has no idea of the normal ratio of quadriceps/hamstrings strength at 60 degrees/second. Lack of specific academic knowledge will result in a candidate not being able to identify the correct answer using a Phase I, Phase II or Phase III approach. However, by applying a Phase IV approach and utilizing deductive reasoning strategies, a candidate can significantly increase his/her chances of identifying the best answer without applying direct academic knowledge.

In this item, the stem asks a candidate to identify a value which would be representative of a normal quadriceps/hamstrings ratio at 60 degrees/second. As with many measurements in physical therapy, precise normal values are difficult to ascertain, and therefore often are expressed in ranges. By applying this knowledge to the examination item, a candidate should be able to eliminate options 3 and 4. Since options 3 and 4 are so close in value they imply each other's incorrectness. Although in this example deductive reasoning strategies were not able to identify the correct answer, they were able to eliminate two of the four possible options. By eliminating the two options, a candidate now has a 50% chance of identifying the best answer, even without utilizing any direct academic or clinical knowledge.

Answer Key

1. Answer: 2   Resource: Pierson (p. 267)
   Question Type: Where
   Content Area: Intervention

   The effect of gravity necessitates the collection bag being positioned below the level of the patient's bladder.

2. Answer: 4   Resource: Currier (p. 265)
   Question Type: Why
   Content Area: Intervention

   Correlation coefficients range from +1.00 to -1.00. Since the question does not ask for a positive or negative correlation, the strongest relationship is indicated by -.89.

3. Answer: 2   Resource: Hamill (p. 236)
   Question Type: Why
   Content Area: Evaluation, Diagnosis, Prognosis, and Outcomes

   A gross estimate of quadriceps:hamstrings ratio is 3:2.

We have attempted to illustrate how the four phase process can be applied to a number of different sample questions. Although candidates may not always be able to identify the correct answer using this strategy, when used appropriately, it can serve as a valuable tool to maximize a candidate's performance on the Physical Therapist Examination.

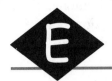

Exercise Three

The following exercise contains ten sample questions for candidates to answer. Resist the urge to approach the questions in a random fashion and instead begin to gain confidence in your ability to answer the questions utilizing the four phase process. An answer key, which is located at the conclusion of the exercise, indicates the best answer, question type, and content category for each of the sample questions.

1. Physical therapists routinely assess the amount of assistance a patient needs to complete a selected activity. Categories of assistance include maximal, moderate, minimal, stand-by or supervision. This type of classification system is most representative of a/an:

    1. interval scale
    2. nominal scale
    3. ordinal scale
    4. ratio scale

2. Chest percussion and vibration are appropriate bronchial drainage techniques for all of the following except the:

    1. anterior apical segment
    2. lingula
    3. left middle lobe
    4. right middle lobe

3. A patient diagnosed with chondromalacia patellae is referred to physical therapy. During the examination, the physical therapist measures the patient's Q angle as 23 degrees bilaterally. Which clinical finding is not typically associated with an increased Q angle?

    1. increased lateral tibial torsion
    2. genu valgum
    3. increased femoral anteversion
    4. patella alta

4. A patient seen twice in physical therapy calls her physical therapist and states that she is no longer interested in therapy and will not return for any additional appointments. The therapist inquires as to the reason for this decision, but the patient refuses to provide any additional information. The therapist's most immediate response should be to:

    1. inform the referring physician of the patient's decision
    2. document the incident in the medical record
    3. call back and ask the patient to reschedule
    4. notify the insurance company of the patient's decision

5. A physical therapist designs a treatment program for a patient with a nasogastric tube. Which of the following activities should be avoided when treating the patient?

    1. ambulatory distances greater than 100 feet
    2. forward bending range of motion exercises of the head and neck
    3. static balance activities in sitting
    4. shoulder flexion and extension resistive exercises

6. A physical therapist performs passive range of motion to the lower extremities of a patient in the medical intensive care unit. While treating the patient, an alarm on one of the monitoring devices sounds. If the therapist is unfamiliar with the particular piece of monitoring equipment, his most immediate response should be to:

    1. contact the patient's referring physician
    2. contact a member of the nursing staff
    3. attempt to locate a switch to disable the monitoring equipment
    4. disregard the alarm and continue with treatment

7. A physical therapist discusses the status of a patient post surgery with a physician. During the discussion the physician cautions the therapist to be alert for any signs or symptoms of pulmonary embolism. Which scenario is most associated with this medical condition?

    1. depleted body electrolytes
    2. excessive systemic insulin
    3. bladder distension
    4. thrombus formation

8. A physical therapist assesses wrist radial and ulnar deviation with a goniometer. When measuring radial and ulnar deviation, the therapist should position the axis of the goniometer over the:

   1. capitate
   3. lunate
   3. trapezium
   4. trapezoid

9. Individual health care organizations have the responsibility to safeguard their patients' medical records. Which of the following situations would require prior consent for the use of a patient's medical records?

   1. financial audits
   2. quality assurance
   3. transfer of records to another health care organization
   4. research where anonymity is preserved

10. While ambulating with a transfemoral prosthesis, a patient demonstrates an abducted gait on the prosthetic side. Which of the following is least likely to cause this type of gait deviation?

   1. tightness of the gluteus medius
   2. discomfort on the adductor longus tendon
   3. the medial wall of the prosthesis is too low
   4. the prosthetic limb is too long

Answer Key

1. Answer: 3   Resource: Best (p. 146)
   Question Type: What/Which
   Content Area: Intervention

   An ordinal scale permits the ranking of items, however the actual difference between adjacent ranks may not be equal.

2. Answer: 3   Resource: Brannon (p. 43)
   Question Type: What/Which
   Content Area: Intervention

   The left lung does not have a middle lobe.

3. Answer: 4   Resource: Magee (p. 729)
   Question Type: What/Which
   Content Area: Examination

   A Q angle less than 20 degrees is significantly above the normal value for males or females. Patella alta is often associated with a diminished Q angle.

4. Answer: 2   Resource: Kettenbach (p. 31)
   Question Type: How/When
   Content Area: Intervention

   It is necessary for the therapist to document the phone conversation in the medical record in a timely fashion.

5. Answer: 2   Resource: Pierson (p. 265)
   Question Type: How/When
   Content Area: Intervention

   A nasogastric tube is a plastic device that is inserted through the nostril and into the stomach. Movements of the head and neck can be disruptive.

6. Answer: 2   Resource: Guide for Professional
                                          Conduct
   Question Type: How/When
   Content Area: Standards of Practice

   Since the therapist is unfamiliar with the monitoring device it is necessary to contact another health care professional. The most accessible and logical choice would be a member of the nursing staff.

7. Answer: 4   Resource: Hillegass (p. 218)
   Question Type: What/Which
   Content Area: Evaluation, Diagnosis, Prognosis, and Outcomes

   A pulmonary embolism results from a blood clot or thrombus that travels from a systemic vein through the right side of the heart into the pulmonary circulation. The blood clot or thrombus eventually lodges in the pulmonary artery or one of its branches.

8. Answer: 1   Resource: Norkin (p. 88)
   Question Type: Where
   Content Area: Examination

   When measuring radial and ulnar deviation, the axis of the goniometer is placed over the middle of the dorsal aspect of the wrist over the capitate.

9. Answer: 3   Resource: Scott-Promoting Legal
   Question Type: What/Which   Awareness (p. 118)
   Content Area: Intervention

   Failure to obtain informed consent from a patient prior to releasing medical records to another organization can be considered malpractice.

10. Answer: 3   Resource: O'Sullivan (p. 666)
    Question Type: Why
    Content Area: Evaluation, Diagnosis, Prognosis, and Outcomes

    A low medial wall would not cause an abducted gait deviation; a high medial wall could be a potential cause.

Recent Developments in Item Construction

There have been a number of changes in item construction on the Physical Therapist Examination within the past few years, most notably the introduction of paired items and graphically enhanced items. Although representing a relatively small percentage of the total examination, candidates need to be comfortable answering each type of item. Both paired items and graphically enhanced items will be incorporated into the remaining exercises.

Paired Items

Paired items consist of general case information followed by two individual items. Candidates need to use the case information to answer each of the items, although the items themselves remain independent. An example of a paired item is as follows:

The following information should be used to answer questions 1 and 2:

A 65-year-old male diagnosed with chronic obstructive pulmonary disease is referred to physical therapy shortly after being admitted to an acute care hospital. The patient reports that he stopped smoking four weeks ago, however denies any improvement in his exercise tolerance. He is extremely frustrated with his present condition and indicates that even the most basic activities have become extremely difficult.

1. As a component of the treatment regime the physical therapist instructs the patient in pursed-lip breathing. The most appropriate duration of inhalation and exhalation is represented by:

   1. 2 second inhalation; 4 second exhalation
   2. 4 second inhalation; 2 second exhalation
   3. 4 second inhalation; 4 second exhalation
   4. 4 second inhalation; 6 second exhalation

2. The physical therapist uses several objective measures to monitor the patient's response to exercise during the session. Which objective measure would be the most appropriate to avoid hypoxemia?

   1. lung volumes and capacities
   2. blood pressure
   3. oxygen saturation rate
   4. blood glucose level

Graphically Enhanced Items

Graphically enhanced items consist of figures, diagrams, pictures, or other static images that are combined with traditional text in an examination item. An example of a graphically enhanced item is as follows:

The following figure should be used to answer question 3:

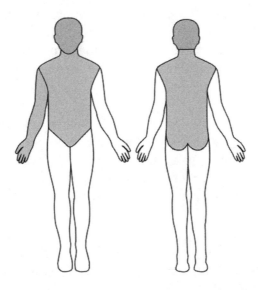

3. A 32-year-old male sustained extensive burns after lighting himself on fire during a suicide attempt. The shaded portion of the body diagrams represent the areas affected by the burns. Using the rule of nines, what percentage of the patient's body was involved?

    1. 40.5%
    2. 44.0%
    3. 49.5%
    4. 54.5%

Answer Key

1. Answer: 4   Resource: Hillegass (p. 736)
   Patients should be instructed to inhale through the nose and exhale through pursed lips in a very slow and methodical manner with exhalation time being greater than inhalation time. The most appropriate duration for pursed-lip breathing is a four second inhalation and a six second exhalation. Potential benefits of pursed-lip breathing include diminished rate of respiration, decreased minute ventilation, and decreased dyspnea.

2. Answer: 3   Resource: Hillegass (p. 665)
   A pulse oximeter can be utilized to monitor a patient's oxygen saturation rate. Hypoxemic states may occur at oxygen saturation levels less than 90%. Modifying the activity level or increasing supplemental oxygen are two methods to address diminished oxygen saturation levels.

3. Answer: 3   Resource: O'Sullivan (p. 852)
   The percentage of the body surface burned in an adult can be calculated using the rule of nines: anterior thorax (18%) + posterior thorax (18%) + head (9%) + anterior arm (4.5%) = 49.5%

Time Constraints

Like many objective examinations, candidates have a specified amount of time to complete the Physical Therapist Examination. For physical therapists, the available time is four and one half hours. Since the examination consists of 225 questions, candidates will have 72 seconds available to answer each question. This number, although correct when viewing the examination as a whole, can be misleading. There will be many questions that a candidate will be able to answer in much less than 72 seconds, whereas other questions will take somewhat longer. The key to success lies in progressing through the examination in a consistent and predictable manner.

Although 72 seconds per question does not seem like a great deal of time, the majority of candidates will have ample time to complete the examination. Despite this fact, it is important to pay attention to the elapsed time during the examination. It also is important to know your test taking history. Are you typically one of the first, one of the last, or somewhere in the middle of individuals completing an examination? This information is important as you plan your test taking strategy.

In order to make sure your pace is appropriate during practice sessions, we suggest placing a small notation in the margin next to question number 50, 100, 150, and 200. When taking the actual Physical Therapist Examination, the same objective can be accomplished by writing the question numbers on a piece of paper and placing it next to the computer. These notations should remind candidates to check on the elapsed time at selected intervals throughout the examination. This technique will allow candidates to assess their progress and modify their pace, if needed. Specific guidelines are difficult to determine; however, in general candidates should answer a minimum of 50 questions an hour.

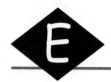

Exercise: Time Management

Candidates will have two hours to complete the following 100 question examination. The allotted time is consistent with the available time per question on the Physical Therapist Examination. Set a timer for two hours and begin the sample examination. Candidates should use a consistent approach when answering each multiple choice question. After completing the exercise, utilize the answer key located at the conclusion of the exercise to determine the number of questions answered correctly. Record your score for the exercise on the Performance Analysis Summary Sheet located in the Appendix.

1. A physical therapist prepares to perform a Lachman test on a patient with a suspected anterior cruciate ligament injury. Why is the Lachman test considered to be more accurate than the anterior drawer test?

   1. hand placement is more difficult in the anterior drawer test
   2. the anterior joint capsule is more lax in the anterior drawer test
   3. the hamstrings pull in direct opposition to the anterior drawer test and often prevent anterior translation of the tibia on the femur
   4. the shape of the menisci allow greater anterior tibial translation in a position emphasizing knee flexion

2. A physical therapist designs an inservice for physical therapy aides to expose them to basic elements associated with superficial heating agents. Which of the following statements regarding hot packs is not accurate?

   1. tissue temperature elevation at depths approaching one centimeter is possible using hot packs
   2. 3-5 towel layers should be used between a hot pack and the patient's skin
   3. hot packs are stored in water at a temperature of approximately 160 degrees Fahrenheit
   4. hot packs do not retain significant amounts of heat for periods greater than 20 minutes

3. A physical therapist participates in a research study that examines the effects of an experimental surgical procedure on selected functional activities in patients with multiple sclerosis. If the study utilizes female patients with ages ranging from 25-45, what type of validity has been most significantly compromised?

    1. construct
    2. external
    3. predictive
    4. content

4. A physical therapist attempts to differentiate closed chain exercise from open chain exercise during a rehabilitation seminar. Which of the following is most representative of a closed chain exercise using the upper extremity?

    1. completing an arm curl using a five pound weight
    2. using the upper extremity during crutch walking
    3. performing an upper extremity D1 flexion pattern
    4. lifting a ten pound weight from the ground to a platform at waist level

5. A physical therapist develops a positioning program for a seven-year-old boy who sustained a head injury in a fall from a tree house. Which of the following would not be a goal of the positioning program?

    1. promote pulmonary hygiene
    2. enhance skin integrity
    3. prevent contractures
    4. facilitate primitive reflexes

6. A physical therapist administers a vapocoolant spray using a spray and stretch technique to treat a patient with trigger points and muscle guarding in the upper trapezius region. Which of the following is the chemical compound most frequently associated with vapocoolant sprays?

    1. ethyl acetate
    2. fluori-methane
    3. ethyl chloride
    4. chlorazene

7. A physical therapist completes an examination on a 46-year-old male with a history of obstructive pulmonary disease. The patient complains of intermittent dyspnea and a persistent cough. Bronchial drainage reveals excessive sputum production that appears to be purulent. The most likely disease classification is:

   1. chronic bronchitis
   2. emphysema
   3. atelectasis
   4. pneumonia

8. A physical therapist attempts to determine whether a selected treatment was effective in increasing range of motion in a group of patients status post total knee replacement. Range of motion measurements were collected using a goniometer. If the research study includes the use of a control group, which statistical technique is the most appropriate to analyze the data?

   1. chi-square
   2. Spearman rho coefficient
   3. t-test
   4. ANOVA

9. A physical therapist instructs a patient with a venous stasis ulcer to use an intermittent pneumatic compression pump. The unit's inflation pressure is set to 40 mm Hg and the treatment time is 120 minutes. What is the recommended ratio of inflation to deflation time?

   1. 1:2
   2. 3:1
   3. 6:1
   4. 1:3

10. The director of physical therapy in an acute care hospital completes a proposed budget for the following fiscal year. As part of the process the director compiles a list of direct and indirect expenses. Which of the following items is an example of an indirect expense?

    1. ultrasound gel
    2. salary of the human resource manager
    3. cost of continuing education for therapists
    4. new equipment purchase

11. A physical therapist passively moves a patient's upper extremity through a selected range of motion while the patient's eyes are closed. The patient then is asked to verbally describe the direction and range of movement of the upper extremity. This technique can be used to examine:

1. barognosis
2. graphesthesia
3. kinesthesia
4. stereognosis

12. A 16-year-old basketball player is anxious to return to athletic competition following rehabilitation from an Achilles tendon rupture. The athlete is objectively ready to return to competition, however continues to demonstrate a severe preoccupation with reinjury. The most appropriate response is to:

1. allow the patient to return to basketball without restriction
2. inform the patient that he should not participate in basketball this season
3. design a functional progression for basketball which allows the patient to progress to higher level activities in a gradual fashion
4. discuss other less demanding athletic activities with the patient

13. A patient rehabilitating from an acute knee injury is examined in physical therapy. The medical record indicates the patient has 0-65 degrees of active and passive motion in the involved knee and moderate effusion. The patient is able to ambulate with a moderate limp and describes pain with prolonged weight bearing. Which special test would be least effective to assess the patient's ligamentous integrity?

1. Lachman test
2. anterior drawer test
3. Varus stress test
4. Losee's test

14. A physical therapist records the vital signs of a 42-year-old male before beginning an exercise program. The therapist determines that the patient's respiration rate and pulse rate are within normal limits. If the therapist expresses the value as a ratio of respiratory rate to pulse rate, which of the following would be considered normal?

1. 1:5
2. 1:3
3. 4:1
4. 6:1

15. A physical therapist identifies several inconsistencies between a patient's subjective complaints and the objective findings of an examination. Which section of a S.O.A.P. note would include a discussion of the identified inconsistencies?

    1. subjective
    2. objective
    3. assessment
    4. plan

16. A patient eight days status post right total hip replacement loses his balance and falls to the ground. The patient is visibly shaken by the fall, but insists that he is uninjured. The physical therapist examines the right hip and although active motion elicits pain, all other findings are inconclusive. The therapist should immediately:

    1. continue with the current treatment so the patient does not focus on the incident
    2. notify the director of rehabilitation about the incident
    3. document the incident and contact a physician to examine the patient
    4. document the incident and gradually resume prior treatment

17. A 21-year-old male suffers a primary anterior dislocation of his right shoulder playing football. The athlete is referred to physical therapy after three weeks of immobilization. A physical therapist might elect to begin treatment with all of the following except:

    1. isometric shoulder exercises
    2. passive range of motion exercises
    3. active assistive range of motion exercises
    4. high speed isokinetic exercises

18. A physical therapist completes an upper extremity goniometric examination. The therapist records right elbow active range of motion as 15 - 0 - 150 degrees. The total available elbow range of motion for this patient is:

    1. 135 degrees
    2. 150 degrees
    3. 165 degrees
    4. 180 degrees

19. A physical therapist conducts a study that measures knee flexion range of motion two weeks following arthroscopic surgery. Assuming a normal distribution, what percentage of patients participating in the study should achieve a goniometric measurement value greater than one standard deviation below the mean?

1. 49%
2. 64%
3. 68%
4. 84%

20. A physical therapist examines a patient with unilateral lower extremity weakness. As the patient performs hip flexion in supine the therapist helps the patient complete the full range of motion. This would best be described as:

1. active exercise
2. passive exercise
3. resistive exercise
4. active assistive exercise

21. A physical therapist performs gait training activities with an eight-year-old child who utilizes a reciprocating gait orthosis. Which medical diagnosis is most often associated with the use of this type of orthotic device?

1. cerebral palsy
2. Down syndrome
3. Legg-Calve-Perthes disease
4. spina bifida

22. A physical therapist employed in an acute care hospital works as a team with a physical therapist assistant. Which of the following would have the greatest impact on how the physical therapist assistant is utilized?

1. the judgment of the supervising physical therapist
2. the length of the formal academic training of the physical therapist assistant
3. the patient population and current hospital census
4. the established productivity standards for physical therapist assistants

23. A physical therapist administers the Tinetti Performance Oriented Mobility Assessment Scale to a patient rehabilitating from a prolonged illness. Which of the following statements most accurately describes this outcome measure?

1. consists of 14 tasks of every day life
2. assesses balance and gait using a 2-3 point ordinal scale
3. designed to measure margin of self-initiated stability
4. examines the ability to modify gait in response to task demands

24. A manager of a developing physical therapy practice negotiates payment terms with a third party payer. The manager proposes to be reimbursed by each increment of service or product provided to patients. This type of payment method is best termed:

1. cost-based payment
2. fee for service payment
3. capitation payment
4. case rate payment

25. A patient returns to physical therapy after being examined by a cardiologist. The patient indicates that the cardiologist prescribed a Holter monitor. The primary purpose for utilizing a Holter monitor is to:

1. identify the location and extent of myocardial ischemia
2. assess cardiac response to increasing workloads
3. evaluate the structure and function of cardiac walls, valves, and chambers
4. evaluate cardiac rhythm and correlate symptoms with activity over time

26. A physical therapist employed by a home health agency often uses newspaper as a barrier when setting down equipment in a patient's home. Which of the following actions would serve as the most acceptable disposal technique for the newspaper?

1. ask the patient to safely dispose of the newspaper
2. place the newspaper in the trash within a patient's home
3. dispose of the newspaper in a biomedical waste bag at the home health agency
4. maintain the newspaper to use as a barrier at a future patient visit

27. A physical therapist reviews a distribution of data arranged using a histogram. The distribution is classified as being negatively skewed. Which of the following descriptions best describes this type of presentation?

1. The mode and the mean are to the left of the median.
2. The mode and mean are to the right of the median.
3. The mean and median are to the left of the mode.
4. The mean and median are to the right of the mode.

28. As part of a research study a physical therapist collects data by administering a survey that requires subjects to respond using a Likert scale. This type of scale is typified by:

1. yes or no responses
2. multiple choice questions
3. rank order questions
4. five or more possible responses

29. A physical therapist discusses the differences between Medicare Part A and Part B with a claims examiner. Which of the following services would not be reimbursed through Part A?

1. inpatient hospital care
2. home health aid
3. hospice care
4. durable medical equipment

30. A physical therapist employed in an outpatient private practice reviews the medical records of patients whose primary insurance is Medicare. What is the most appropriate timeframe associated with physician recertification?

1. 30 days
2. 60 days
3. 90 days
4. 120 days

31. A patient recovering from a traumatic brain injury is screened for inclusion in a formal rehabilitation program. Which of the following situations would most prohibit the patient from being involved in the rehabilitation program?

   1. inability to sit supported for 60 minutes
   2. inability to perform self-care activities
   3. maximal assistance required for all transfers
   4. medically unstable

32. A physical therapist completes ambulation activities with a patient rehabilitating from a total hip replacement. Later while documenting in the medical record, the therapist realizes she has exceeded the patient's prescribed weight bearing status. The most immediate therapist action is to:

   1. disregard the incident since the patient did not report any discomfort
   2. discuss the situation with the director of rehabilitation
   3. inform the orthopedic surgeon of the incident
   4. complete an incident report

33. A patient is unable to actively participate during a transfer and as a result requires a two man lift to be moved into bed. The most appropriate documentation of transfer status is:

   1. the patient requires maximal assistance for transfers
   2. the patient requires maximal assistance of two for transfers
   3. the patient is dependent requiring a two man lift transfer
   4. the patient requires moderate assistance using a two man lift transfer

34. A physical therapist examines a patient status post CVA at bedside. The patient is unable to move without assistance. The therapist's highest priority should be:

   1. toilet transfers
   2. positioning
   3. gait analysis
   4. cognitive assessment

35. A patient two weeks status post CVA exhibits hypertonicity in his hemiplegic upper extremity. All of the following would be indicated as treatment except:

   1. use of a sling
   2. active assistive exercise
   3. passive range of motion
   4. weight bearing techniques

36. A patient with chronic venous insufficiency presents with significant edema in the lower extremities. Which treatment option would be the most appropriate for the initial visit?

   1. intermittent compression and patient education
   2. custom fitted stockings
   3. intermittent compression and warm whirlpool
   4. instruction in a lower extremity exercise program

37. A physical therapist completes a research study that examines the relationship between elbow position and grip strength. The most important action to benefit the field of physical therapy is to:

   1. describe the design procedures in sufficient detail
   2. disseminate the results of the research study
   3. develop additional ideas for future research
   4. identify how the research study relates to the current body of knowledge

38. A patient recently involved in a motor vehicle accident is referred to physical therapy after being diagnosed with a cervical strain. During the examination the physical therapist palpates the anterior aspect of the neck. Which of the following bony structures is most superior?

   1. thyroid cartilage
   2. first cricoid ring
   3. hyoid bone
   4. C5 vertebral body

39. A patient rehabilitating from a fractured humerus develops a resultant musculocutaneous nerve lesion. Which objective finding is most indicative of musculocutaneous nerve involvement?

    1. weakness of shoulder medial rotation
    2. sensory loss in the lateral forearm
    3. winging of the inferior angle of the scapula
    4. loss of contour in the shoulder due to deltoid paralysis

40. A patient diagnosed with Erb-Duchenne palsy is referred to physical therapy. The medical record indicates the patient sustained the injury at birth. Which of the following objective findings would not be expected based on the patient's diagnosis?

    1. paralysis of the biceps and brachialis
    2. absent sensation in the deltoid region
    3. absent biceps and brachioradialis reflex
    4. paralysis of the intrinsic hand muscles

41. A physical therapist develops a plan of care for a 47-year-old male rehabilitating from a low back injury. As part of the plan of care the therapist assists the patient with hamstrings stretching exercises. According to the disablement model, which level is this particular intervention directed toward?

    1. pathology
    2. impairment
    3. functional limitation
    4. disability

42. The director of rehabilitation services summarizes various third party payment methods with members of an administrative task force. Which of the following methods allows providers to maximize income when fewer patients receive services?

    1. cost-based payment
    2. per diem payment
    3. case rate payment
    4. capitation payment

43. A physical therapist participates in a community presentation designed to promote breast cancer awareness. As part of the presentation, the therapist discusses mammography guidelines for individuals over 50 years of age. Which of the following would be the most appropriate frequency for a mammogram?

1. once a year
2. once every three years
3. once every five years
4. once every seven years

44. A physical therapist treats a patient on the neonatal intensive care unit. The therapist should adhere to all of the following guidelines when treating the neonate except:

1. recognize the impact of physiological stress on the neonate
2. assist with parent-infant interaction
3. perform positioning and daily care activities with as little handling as possible
4. allow for periods of rest during treatment

45. A physical therapist attempts to determine the percent body fat of a patient using an objective measure. Which of the following measures would be least appropriate to meet the stated objective?

1. hydrostatic weighing
2. skinfold measurements
3. body mass index
4. bioimpedance

46. A physical therapist employed in a rehabilitation hospital participates in a weekly team meeting for a patient diagnosed with a traumatic brain injury. During the meeting each member of the rehabilitation team (physical therapist, occupational therapist, speech therapist, nurse, dietician) describes the patient's progress toward meeting established goals and attempts to identify any relevant barriers to progress. This type of team is best termed a/an:

1. unidisciplinary team
2. multidisciplinary team
3. interdisciplinary team
4. transdisciplinary team

47. A physical therapist is involved in a research study that examines the effect of aerobic exercise on body composition. The research study uses selected skinfold measurements at 30 day intervals to identify changes in body composition. The measurement procedure requires the therapist to take duplicate measures at each site and retest if the measurements are not within an acceptable margin of error. Which of the following consecutive values would be considered within the acceptable margin of error?

1. 2.0 cm and 2.5 cm
2. 1.8 cm and 1.5 cm
3. 28 mm and 30 mm
4. 54 mm and 48 mm

48. A physical therapist works on transfer activities with a patient diagnosed with a complete C5 spinal cord injury. Which of the following muscles would the patient be able to utilize during the training session?

1. brachioradialis
2. pronator teres
3. extensor carpi radialis brevis
4. latissimus dorsi

49. Prior to performing a manual muscle test of the anterior deltoid, a patient is asked to perform active shoulder flexion. The patient is able to actively move the extremity from 0-160 degrees of shoulder flexion. Assuming the cause of the limitation is due to a capsular restriction, what is the most appropriate method when testing the anterior deltoid?

1. perform the manual muscle test in a horizontal plane
2. perform the manual muscle test with gravity-eliminated
3. perform the manual muscle test against gravity
4. avoid performing the manual muscle test due to the limitation in range of motion

50. A physical therapist classifies a patient's posture as lordotic after completing a postural assessment. Which muscle group would you expect to be shortened based on the results of the postural assessment?

1. intercostals
2. hip flexors
3. scapula retractors
4. abdominals

51. A physical therapist completes a series of resisted tests on a patient referred to physical therapy with a lower extremity injury. During the testing the patient indicates that he begins to experience pain after a number of repetitions. The most likely explanation is:

   1. a complete tendon rupture
   2. capsular laxity
   3. intermittent claudication
   4. emotional hypersensitivity

52. A clinical instructor demonstrates a mobilization technique for a student. The clinical instructor describes the movement as a large amplitude oscillation that does not reach the limit of the range. This description is most representative of:

   1. grade I
   2. grade II
   3. grade III
   4. grade IV

53. An administrator in a rehabilitation hospital presents an inservice on legal and ethical issues for health care practitioners. During the inservice the administrator reviews several types of law that affect the health care system. Which type of law is based on court judgments, decisions, and decrees?

   1. constitutional law
   2. statutory law
   3. common law
   4. administrative law

54. A physical therapist examines a patient's sputum sample. The therapist describes the color of the sample as yellow. Which condition is most likely associated with a yellow sputum sample?

   1. pulmonary edema
   2. neoplasm
   3. infection
   4. pneumonia

55. A physician note indicates that a patient exhibits dysdiadochokinesia. The most appropriate test to assess dysdiadochokinesia is:

1. heel on shin
2. alternating finger to nose
3. deep tendon reflexes
4. passive movement

56. A physical therapist observes that a number of physical therapy aides often jeopardize patient safety when performing selected transfers. The most immediate intervention is to:

1. offer to assist physical therapy aides with selected transfers
2. prohibit physical therapy aides from performing selected transfers
3. develop a formal training session on appropriate transfer techniques
4. provide written literature which outlines basic transfer techniques

57. A patient rehabilitating from a motor vehicle accident complains that his pain medication is overdue. The most appropriate therapist action is to:

1. administer the patient's pain medication
2. ask the patient to focus on the treatment session and not the pain
3. notify the nursing staff of the patient's complaint
4. document the patient's complaint in the medical record

58. A 63-year-old male is referred to physical therapy after being diagnosed with Parkinson's disease. Which of the following should be given the highest priority during the initial session?

1. introducing the patient to other patients with Parkinson's disease
2. determining the patient's educational background and general knowledge
3. explaining to the patient the role of the physical therapist
4. determining the patient's current functional status

59. A patient in an acute care hospital attempts to get out of bed in preparation for ambulation activities. The patient has not been able to ambulate since being admitted to the hospital four weeks ago. The most immediate physical therapist action is to:

    1. disconnect the patient's intravenous line
    2. provide a straight cane for ambulation activities
    3. have the patient sit on the edge of the bed with his feet on the floor
    4. instruct family members in various transfer techniques

60. A physical therapist performs daily goniometric measurements on a patient status post total knee arthroplasty. To ensure the most reliable goniometric measurement, the therapist should:

    1. utilize the same goniometer for each measurement
    2. accurately identify appropriate bony landmarks
    3. perform goniometric measurements at the same time each day
    4. provide the patient with concise and explicit verbal instructions

61. A physical therapist observes a patient with Parkinson's disease complete a series of functional activities. The therapist notes that the patient has difficulty initiating movement and is slow to carry out a task once it has begun. This type of movement pattern is best termed:

    1. akinesia
    2. hypokinesia
    3. bradykinesia
    4. hyperkinesia

62. A physical therapist completes a series of examination procedures in order to assess an infant's primitive reflexes. When assessing the Moro reflex, what is the most appropriate stimulus?

    1. touch the skin along the spine from the shoulder to the hip
    2. turn the head to one side
    3. head suddenly dropping into extension
    4. loud and sudden noise

63. A physical therapist attempts to assess the L5 myotome in a patient with peripheral neuropathy. The most appropriate muscle to assess is the:

1. iliopsoas
2. gastrocnemius
3. extensor hallucis longus
4. plantar interossei

64. A physical therapist administers the Mini-Mental State Examination to a 57-year-old female recently admitted to the hospital following a motor vehicle accident. Which of the following commands would be the most appropriate to assess orientation?

1. repeat the name of three objects that were mentioned earlier
2. count backwards by seven beginning with the number 100
3. ask the patient the current month, date, and year
4. copy a given design using paper and pencil

65. A physical therapist completes a developmental assessment on a seven-month-old infant. Assuming normal development, which milestone would the child most likely be able to perform?

1. creeps on hands and feet
2. walks along furniture
3. crawl backwards
4. bends over in standing to look between the legs

66. A physical therapist working in an acute care hospital often utilizes a gait belt when working on ambulation activities with patients. Which of the following is the most appropriate action?

1. utilize a protective barrier over clothing at all times when using the gait belt
2. clean the gait belt once per month unless the belt is soiled with body fluid
3. clean the gait belt after each patient use
4. clean the gait belt only when it makes direct contact with the patient's skin

67. A physical therapist employed in an acute care hospital treats a patient diagnosed with liver disease. The therapist notes that the patient's skin and eyes appear to have a yellow tint. Which of the following conditions is most consistent with this type of clinical presentation?

    1. human immunodeficiency virus
    2. hepatitis
    3. tuberculosis
    4. meningitis

68. A physical therapist performs cardiopulmonary resuscitation with a colleague on a 28-year-old male that collapsed in the waiting room. When performing CPR, the most appropriate ratio of compressions to breaths is:

    1. 1:5
    2. 5:1
    3. 15:2
    4. 2:15

69. A physical therapist would like to use ultrasound as a component of a patient's plan of care, but is concerned about the potential of the modality to exacerbate the patient's current inflammation. The most effective method to address the therapist's concern is:

    1. utilize ultrasound with a frequency of 1 MHz
    2. limit treatment time to five minutes
    3. incorporate a pulsed 20% duty cycle
    4. select an ultrasound intensity less than 1.5 W/cm^2

70. A patient positioned in prone on a treatment plinth complains of pain in the low back. In order to alleviate the pain, the physical therapist attempts to reduce the patient's lumbar lordosis. The most appropriate modification is:

    1. place a pillow under the patient's upper or middle chest
    2. place a pillow under the patient's lower abdomen
    3. place a pillow lengthwise from the patient's pelvis to the thorax
    4. place a small bolster under the patient's anterior ankles

71. A physical therapist attempts to assess the chest mobility of a patient diagnosed with chronic obstructive pulmonary disease. To assess lower lobe expansion the therapist should:

   1. place the tips of the thumbs along the manubrium and extend the fingers laterally around the ribs
   2. place the tips of the thumbs at the midsternal line at the sternal notch and extend the fingers above the clavicles
   3. place the tips of the thumbs at the xiphoid process and extend the fingers laterally around the ribs
   4. place the tips of the thumbs along the patient's back at the spinous processes of T10 - T12 and extend the fingers around the ribs

72. A patient rehabilitating from a CVA exhibits signs and symptoms of depression. Which of the following is not representative of a patient with depression?

   1. the patient develops unrealistic rehabilitation goals
   2. the patient exhibits decreased participation in physical therapy
   3. the patient expresses feelings of worthlessness
   4. the patient exhibits periods of agitation and loss of energy

73. A physical therapist completes an examination on a patient referred to physical therapy with a cervical strain. During the examination the therapist begins to suspect there may be a lesion interfering with neural conduction. Which resisted test would supply the therapist with information on the C4 myotome?

   1. elbow extension
   2. shoulder abduction
   3. shoulder shrug
   4. elbow flexion

74. A physical therapist completes a manual muscle test of the flexor digitorum brevis. In order to accurately assess the strength of the muscle, the therapist should apply pressure against the:

   1. dorsal surface of the middle phalanx of the four toes in the direction of extension
   2. plantar surface of the middle phalanx of the four toes in the direction of extension
   3. dorsal surface of the distal phalanx of the four toes in the direction of extension
   4. plantar surface of the distal phalanx of the four toes in the direction of extension

75. A physical therapist attempts to identify an appropriate statistical test to analyze a set of data. What type of measurement scale is necessary when using a parametric statistical test?

1. nominal or ordinal
2. ordinal or interval
3. nominal or interval
4. interval or ratio

76. A 72-year-old male status post CVA is referred to physical therapy. The patient is able to ambulate independently and has good upper extremity strength, however is unable to communicate through verbal or written means. This type of deficit is best termed:

1. apraxia
2. aphasia
3. aphonia
4. aplasia

77. As part of a quality assurance program, a physical therapy department embarks on an outcome assessment study. When working with outcome assessment the most critical period of time is:

1. at the conclusion of a selected treatment session
2. at the conclusion of care in relation to the goals of treatment
3. at the conclusion of a 14 day period
4. after a scheduled physician visit

78. A patient is diagnosed with a bacterial infection shortly after being admitted to the hospital. Which of the following laboratory tests would you expect to be most affected based on the patient's diagnosis?

1. platelet count
2. hemoglobin
3. hematocrit
4. white blood cell count

79. A physical therapist examines a patient referred to physical therapy with low back pain. During the examination the therapist determines that the patient is restricted in a capsular pattern at the hip. Which of the following motions would you expect to be limited at the hip?

1. flexion and extension
2. abduction and medial rotation
3. adduction and lateral rotation
4. abduction and extension

80. A patient scheduled to undergo thoracic surgery is given preoperative instructions. During the training session the patient seems very discouraged and anxious about the impending surgery. The most appropriate mechanism to offer emotional support is to:

1. tell the patient he will do just fine
2. notify family members of the patient's present state
3. visit the patient immediately after surgery
4. listen to the patient express his feelings

81. A physical therapist employed in an outpatient physical therapy clinic treats a 32-year-old male diagnosed with trochanteric bursitis. During the treatment session the patient asks the therapist if it is possible to view his medical record. The most appropriate therapist action is to:

1. attempt to secure approval from the referring physician
2. ask the patient to sign a "hold harmless" form prior to examining the medical record
3. arrange a mutually acceptable time to allow the patient to review the medical record
4. instruct the patient that established confidentiality standards do not permit the patient to review the medical record

82. A physical therapist named in a lawsuit deliberately shreds several physical therapy records related to pending litigation. The legal term most consistent with this situation is:

1. vicarious liability
2. malpractice
3. libel
4. spoliation

83. A physical therapist employed in a home health agency arrives at the home of a 75-year-old male. After knocking on the door for several minutes it becomes apparent that the patient is not at home. In a subsequent conversation, the patient indicates that he routinely goes out to lunch with his friends. The most appropriate therapist action based on the patient's comment is to:

    1. continue providing home health services under Medicare Part A
    2. attempt to have home health services covered through Medicare Part B
    3. remind the patient that he must stay at home if he is going to qualify for Medicare Part A
    4. refer the patient to outpatient physical therapy services

84. A patient describes his typical sleeping position as lying on his stomach with his arms by his side. Which bony prominence would be most susceptible to a pressure injury in this position?

    1. posterior iliac crest
    2. occipital tuberosity
    3. medial epicondyle of the humerus
    4. anterior portion of the head of the humerus

85. A physical therapist covering for a colleague on vacation reviews the parameters of a recent electrical stimulation treatment session using alternating current. Which of the following parameters would not be used to describe this type of current?

    1. amplitude
    2. frequency
    3. interpulse interval
    4. phase duration

86. A physical therapist attempts to develop a research manuscript after completing a research study. When drafting the manuscript the therapist reports the statistical findings of the research study. In which section of the manuscript should this type of reporting occur?

    1. methods
    2. results
    3. discussion
    4. conclusion

87. A physical therapy manager is informed by the Director of Rehabilitation that beginning next week the department must provide physical therapy services on Sunday. The manager is concerned that the staff will not be receptive to the idea and as a result schedules a department meeting. The most immediate action to meet the staffing need is:

1. ask for volunteers to work during the expanded time
2. develop a questionnaire to determine how other physical therapy departments meet their staffing needs
3. appoint a committee to develop options to meet the staffing needs
4. ask the Director of Rehabilitation to reconsider the need for the expanded coverage

88. A physical therapist uses infrared radiation as a form of superficial heat to treat a patient with arthritis. The therapist begins the treatment session with the infrared lamp 45 centimeters away from the target area. If the therapist later elects to move the lamp 90 centimeters away from the target area, what percentage of the original radiation intensity has been maintained?

1. 25%
2. 33%
3. 50%
4. 75%

89. A physical therapist reviews an entry in the medical record that indicates a 29-year-old male has normal dorsiflexion range of motion. Which measurement would be considered within normal limits?

1. 0 degrees dorsiflexion
2. 0-3 degrees dorsiflexion
3. 0-8 degrees dorsiflexion
4. 0-17 degrees dorsiflexion

90. A physical therapist assists a patient rehabilitating from shoulder surgery with Codman's pendulum exercises. While performing the exercises the patient begins to experience back pain. The most appropriate modified patient position would be:

1. supine
2. standing
3. sidelying
4. prone

91. A patient diagnosed with chronic venous insufficiency is referred to physical therapy. After evaluating the patient, the physical therapist's general treatment goal is to increase venous return and reduce edema. Which of the following would not be part of the expected plan of care?

    1. manual massage of the extremities in a proximal to distal direction
    2. use of an intermittent compression pump
    3. avoid prolonged periods of static standing and sitting with the legs in a dependent position
    4. elevation of the foot of the bed during rest

The following figure should be used to answer question 92:

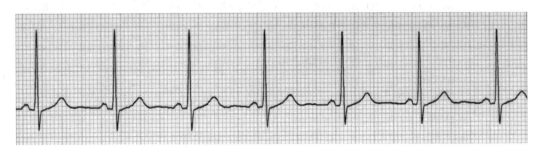

92. A patient is required to have an electrocardiogram as part of a physical examination. A rhythm strip from the electrocardiogram while the patient was at rest is displayed above. Assuming the patient's heart rate was determined to be 70 beats per minute, the heart rate is most representative of:

    1. sinus bradycardia
    2. normal sinus rhythm
    3. sinus arrhythmia
    4. sinus tachycardia

93. A physical therapist teaches a patient with limited shoulder range of motion a self-mobilization technique. The therapist instructs the patient to sit on a firm table and grasp his fingers under the edge of the table. The patient is then asked to lean his trunk away from the stabilized arm. This type of self-mobilization technique can be used to facilitate:

    1. flexion
    2. medial rotation
    3. lateral rotation
    4. abduction

94. A 65-year-old female rehabilitating from a motor vehicle accident is referred to therapy for treatment of lymphedema. Which of the following would not be part of the expected plan of care?

1. application of local heat
2. isometric and isotonic pumping exercises of the distal muscles
3. elevation of the extremity above the level of the heart
4. intermittent mechanical compression

95. A physical therapist examines a 55-year-old male whose subjective complaints include asymmetric pain in the knees and hips. The patient describes the intensity of the pain in proportion to the amount of daily activity. The patient indicates he has been employed as a roofer for the past 20 years. Which disease category is most consistent with this case?

1. systemic lupus erythematosus
2. osteoarthritis
3. rheumatoid arthritis
4. gout

96. A team of health care professionals develops a rehabilitation management program for a patient recovering from a traumatic brain injury. Which of the following steps would be the last to occur?

1. develop long-term rehabilitation goals with the patient and family
2. develop short-term goals and treatment priorities
3. identify significant impairments and disabilities
4. identify tasks and activities that the patient expects to resume

97. A physical therapist administers the Fugl-Meyer Assessment to patients status post CVA in an attempt to identify individuals that may benefit from inclusion in a formal rehabilitation program. What is the primary weakness of this standardized instrument?

1. poor sensitivity
2. time consuming
3. low sensitivity
4. poor theoretical rationale

98. A physical therapist screens a patient status post CVA for placement in a formal rehabilitation program. The patient is medically stable, however needs 24 hour per day monitoring and moderate assistance with mobility and activities of daily living. The patient is presently able to tolerate intense rehabilitation three hours per day. The most appropriate setting for continued therapy is:

    1. an inpatient rehabilitation hospital
    2. a nursing facility
    3. home care
    4. an acute care hospital

99. A patient diagnosed with a grade I anterior talofibular ligament sprain is referred to physical therapy. The best indicator of the patient's expected functional status following rehabilitation would be based on:

    1. the patient's previous functional status
    2. the number of physical therapy visits
    3. the quality of the physical therapy services
    4. the patient's willingness to complete a home exercise program

100. A patient rehabilitating from congestive heart failure is examined in physical therapy. During the examination the patient begins to complain of pain. The most immediate physical therapist action is to:

    1. notify the nursing staff to administer pain medication
    2. contact the referring physician
    3. discontinue the session
    4. ask the patient to describe the location and severity of the pain

Answer Key

1. Answer: 3   Resource: Reider (p. 230)
   The anterior drawer test is performed with the patient in supine with 90 degrees of knee flexion. The examiner grasps the tibia just below the joint line and pulls the tibia forward. In addition to the hamstrings' ability to mask anterior translation of the tibia, patients normally have considerable laxity in the test position (90 degrees of knee flexion).

2. Answer: 2   Resource: Cameron (p. 309)
   Hot packs should be wrapped in 6-8 layers of dry towels. Hot pack covers often account for 2-3 layers depending on the thickness.

3. Answer: 2   Resource: Currier (p. 211)
   External validity refers to the degree that the researcher can generalize from the sample to a larger population. Since the study utilized females with ages ranging from 25-45, external validity would be somewhat compromised.

4. Answer: 2   Resource: Kisner (p. 92)
   Closed chain exercises require that the body moves on a distal segment that is fixed or stable.

5. Answer: 4   Resource: O'Sullivan (p. 187)
   Primitive or tonic reflexes are often present during gestation or infancy before being integrated by the central nervous system. The asymmetrical tonic neck reflex and symmetrical tonic neck reflex are examples of primitive reflexes. Most primitive or tonic reflexes interfere with isolated movement and overall function.

6. Answer: 2   Resource: Cameron (p. 143)
   Fluori-methane is the most commonly utilized vapocoolant spray since it is non-flammable and does not result in excessive temperature reductions in the cutaneous area. Vapocoolant sprays are most commonly utilized to treat trigger points.

7. Answer: 1   Resource: Pauls (p. 601)
   Chronic bronchitis is an obstructive disease characterized by increased mucus secretion of the tracheobronchial tree. Postural drainage techniques and breathing exercises can serve to clear secretions and improve ventilation. Atelectasis and pneumonia are more representative of restrictive pulmonary conditions.

8. Answer: 3   Resource: Currier (p. 252)
The t-test is a statistical procedure for comparing a mean with a norm or comparing two means. The test should not be used for comparing means of more than two groups.

9. Answer: 2   Resource: Cameron (p. 262)
A 3:1 ratio of inflation to deflation is typically recommended when using an intermittent pneumatic compression pump. The deflation period is necessary to allow for venous refilling after compression.

10. Answer: 2   Resource: Walter (p. 265)
A direct expense is typically associated with the production of goods or services. Since the physical therapy department is part of a larger organization the salary of a human resource manager would be considered a shared overhead expense or indirect expense.

11. Answer: 3   Resource: Anderson (p. 957)
Kinesthesia is defined as the ability to perceive extent, direction or weight of movement.

12. Answer: 3   Resource: Shamus (p. 363)
The treatment plan should allow the patient to gradually gain confidence in his ability to return to athletic competition while at the same time have the opportunity to perform sport specific skills.

13. Answer: 2   Resource: Reider (p. 230)
The patient's limitation in active and passive range of motion would make it impossible to perform the anterior drawer test. The anterior drawer test is performed with the patient in supine with 90 degrees of knee flexion.

14. Answer: 1   Resource: Minor (p. 39)
Although normal values deviate from source to source, broad ranges of normal values for respiration rate and heart rate are as follows: respiration rate 12-18 breaths/minute, heart rate 60-100 beats per minute.

15. Answer: 3   Resource: Kettenbach (p. 110)
The assessment section of a S.O.A.P. note provides a platform for a therapist to express his/her professional judgment.

16. Answer: 3   Resource: Guide for Professional
                                                      Conduct
Since the patient is status post total hip replacement it is necessary for the patient to be examined by a physician. The incident must also be documented in the medical record.

17. Answer: 4   Resource: Kisner (p. 352)
High speed isokinetic exercises would be an inappropriate treatment option based on the patient's current status.

18. Answer: 3   Resource: Norkin (p. 26)
Since the 15 is to the left of 0 it is indicative of hyperextension, therefore $150 + 15 = 165$ degrees.

19. Answer: 4   Resource: Best (p. 221)
A normal distribution produces a bell shaped curve where predictable percentages of the population can be determined. 50% of the population falls on each side of the mean and 34% of the population falls between -1 standard deviation and the mean (50% +34% = 84%).

20. Answer: 4   Resource: Minor (p. 134)
Active assistive exercise requires movement performed by a patient with additional movement or mechanical assistance.

21. Answer: 4   Resource: Campbell – Decision Making
                                                      (p. 212)
A reciprocating gait orthosis is a type of hip-knee-ankle orthosis that incorporates a cable connecting the two hip joint mechanisms. The orthosis is most commonly utilized with children diagnosed with spina bifida.

22. Answer: 1   Resource: Guide to Physical Therapist
                                                      Practice (p. S32)
The physical therapist of record is directly responsible for the actions of the physical therapist assistant and therefore it is the judgment of the physical therapist that should primarily determine how the physical therapist assistant is utilized.

23. Answer: 2   Resource: Physical Therapist's Clinical
                                                      Companion (p. 123)
The Tinetti Performance Oriented Mobility Assessment Scale is used to screen patients and identify if there is an increased risk for falling. The first section assesses balance through various functional activities. The second section assesses gait at normal speed and at a rapid, but safe speed. The tool has a combined maximum total of 28 with the risk of falling increasing as the total score decreases.

24. Answer: 2   Resource: Curtis (p. 21)
A fee for service reimbursement model occurs when health care providers are paid for each discrete increment of service or product provided to a patient. The fee schedule is based on what is usual, customary, and reasonable. This model provides enrollees with greater freedom of choice and enhanced access to specialty providers.

25. Answer: 4   Resource: Anderson (p. 823)
    A Holter monitor is a portable unit that records electrocardiograph recordings during activities of daily living. While wearing the monitor patients are responsible for keeping a daily activity log.

26. Answer: 2   Resource: Anemaet (p. 21)
    A newspaper can serve as an effective barrier to prevent the transmission of infectious material. Once the newspaper has been used as a barrier it should be immediately discarded by the physical therapist. Although disposing of the newspaper in a biomedical waste bag may seem like a viable alternative it would be inappropriate to transport the newspaper back to the home health agency.

27. Answer: 3   Resource: Triola (p. 69)
    Skewness refers to the degree of asymmetry to one side of the histogram when compared to the other. Negatively skewed (to the left) is characterized by the mean and median being to the left of the mode.

28. Answer: 4   Resource: Domholdt (p. 207)
    A Likert scale is typically scored on a 5-7 point range indicating a subject's level of agreement with an item. Often a scale value is placed on each of the responses. For example strongly agree = 5; agree = 4; undecided = 3; disagree = 2; strongly disagree = 1.

29. Answer: 4   Resource: Curtis (p. 19)
    Medicare Part A typically covers inpatient hospital stays, skilled nursing facilities, hospice, and short-term care at home due to an illness for which the patient was hospitalized. Durable medical equipment is most often covered through Medicare Part B.

30. Answer: 1   Resource: Nosse (p. 167)
    Medicare requires physician recertification of the patient's treatment plan every 30 days in an outpatient setting.

31. Answer: 4   Resource: O'Sullivan (p. 540)
    Participation in a formal inpatient rehabilitation program requires a minimum of three hours of services from physical therapy, occupational therapy, and speech. Failure to be medically stable would prohibit this type of participation.

32. Answer: 4   Resource: Scott-Promoting Legal
                                                   Awareness (p. 134)
    An incident report should be completed which describes the details of the event in question.

33. Answer: 3   Resource: Kettenbach (p. 49)
The most appropriate form of documentation describes the type of transfer and the amount of assistance necessary to complete the transfer.

34. Answer: 2   Resource: Minor (p. 116)
Positioning should be the therapist's highest priority in order to avoid contractures and tissue breakdown.

35. Answer: 1   Resource: Davies (p. 212)
The use of a sling is not indicated in the treatment of hypertonicity since it will serve to immobilize the arm and reinforce a flexor synergy pattern.

36. Answer: 1   Resource: Kisner (p. 718)
The primary goal of treatment is to increase venous return and reduce edema. Intermittent compression will assist with this goal and patient education will be directed toward decreasing dependent edema.

37. Answer: 2   Resource: Currier (p. 321)
Disseminating the results of a research study is the primary means of expanding the profession's body of knowledge.

38. Answer: 3   Resource: Hoppenfeld (p. 106)
The hyoid bone is located at the same level as the C3 vertebral body. The thyroid cartilage is directly below the hyoid bone.

39. Answer: 2   Resource: Magee (p. 290)
In addition to sensory loss in the lateral forearm, an injury to the musculocutaneous nerve can result in loss of elbow flexion, shoulder forward flexion, and decreased supination.

40. Answer: 4   Resource: Pauls (p. 413)
The intrinsic muscles of the hand are primarily innervated by the C8-T1 nerve roots. Erb-Duchenne palsy is an upper brachial plexus injury typically involving the C5-C6 nerve roots.

41. Answer: 2   Resource: Guide to Physical Therapist
                                                                  Practice (p. S22)
An impairment is defined as a loss or abnormality of physiological, psychological, or anatomical structure or function.

42. Answer: 4   Resource: Curtis (p. 22)
Reimbursement via capitation is based on a per member, per month fee that does not fluctuate based on the amount or frequency of services provided. As a result, when fewer patient services are received the provider maintains the same level of income without incurring additional patient related expenses.

43. Answer: 1   Resource: Bickley (p. 304)
The American Cancer Society recommends that women over 40 years of age have a clinical breast examination and mammography on an annual basis. Other sources indicate that women over 50 years of age should have a mammogram every one to two years.

44. Answer: 3   Resource: Tecklin (p. 91)
Therapeutic handling techniques promote postural alignment and influence normal patterns of movement. Proper therapeutic handling has many benefits and should not be restricted when working with the neonate.

45. Answer: 3   Resource: American College of Sports
                                                    Medicine (p. 63)
Body mass index (BMI) is used to assess weight relative to height, however it is not used to assess percent body fat since it does not consider fat-free density and skeletal mass.

46. Answer: 3   Resource: Ozer (p. 76)
An interdisciplinary team includes several different members of the rehabilitation team that function independently, however routinely report to each other through formal and informal mechanisms and may coordinate care activities. A multidisciplinary team includes several different members of the rehabilitation team, however there is less interaction between team members and communication is primarily through formal channels such as the medical record.

47. Answer: 3   Resource: American College of Sports
                                                    Medicine (p. 65)
Acceptable margin of error when conducting skinfold measurements is 1-2 mm.

48. Answer: 1   Resource: Kendall (p. 266)
The brachioradialis is innervated by the radial nerve (C5-C6) and therefore would be partially innervated in a patient with C5 tetraplegia. The muscle's primary action is to flex the elbow joint.

49. Answer: 3   Resource: Kendall (p. 275)
The patient's limitation in range of motion is due to a capsular restriction and not muscle weakness. As a result it is appropriate to test the muscle against gravity. A horizontal plane and gravity eliminated are synonymous terms in this situation.

50. Answer: 2   Resource: Kendall (p. 106)
A lordotic posture refers to an excessive anterior curve of the lumbar spine resulting in increased anterior pelvic tilt and hip flexion. As a result, a lordotic posture is often associated with shortened hip flexors.

51. Answer: 3   Resource: Kisner (p. 710)
    Insufficient blood supply to an exercising muscle or group of muscles can result in intermittent claudication.

52. Answer: 2   Resource: Kisner (p. 224)
    Grade II oscillations are defined as large amplitude within the range, not reaching the limit.

53. Answer: 3   Resource: Scott-Promoting Legal
                                                     Awareness (p. 5)
    Common law develops over time based on judicial decisions. It is also referred to as judge-made case law.

54. Answer: 3   Resource: Rothstein (p. 533)
    Yellow or greenish sputum is commonly associated with acute or chronic infection.

55. Answer: 2   Resource: Umphred (p. 724)
    Dysdiadochokinesia is the inability to perform rapid alternating movements usually due to cerebellar dysfunction. Asking a patient to point his/her finger to the tip of the nose with reasonable speed and accuracy is a test used to confirm the presence of this condition.

56. Answer: 2   Resource: Standards of Practice
    The physical therapy aides should not be permitted to perform transfers until a remediation plan is developed and implemented.

57. Answer: 3   Resource: Guide for Professional
                                                     Conduct
    The nursing staff is the appropriate party to assess the veracity of the patient's complaint and administer the pain medication if needed.

58. Answer: 4   Resource: O'Sullivan (p. 760)
    By assessing the patient's functional status the therapist will be able to gain valuable information necessary to design a comprehensive plan of care. It will also provide the therapist with a means to assess the future progress and performance of the patient.

59. Answer: 3   Resource: Goodman – Pathology
                                                     (p. 296)
    Since the patient has not ambulated for a significant amount of time, it is advisable to assist him/her to a sitting position as an intermediate step before progressing to standing. This action will minimize the possibility of the patient feeling light headed, dizzy, or exhibiting signs of postural hypotension.

60. Answer: 2   Resource: Norkin (p. 35)
Although each of the options has an influence on the reliability of goniometric measurements, identifying the appropriate bony landmarks is fundamental to any goniometric measurement.

61. Answer: 3   Resource: O'Sullivan (p. 161)
Bradykinesia is defined as extreme slowness of movement. Patients with Parkinson's disease often exhibit bradykinesia, festinating gait, and tremors.

62. Answer: 3   Resource: Ratliffe (p. 266)
The Moro reflex is stimulated by the head dropping into extension suddenly for a few inches resulting in the infant's arms abducting with fingers open followed by the arms crossing the trunk into adduction. The reflex is similar to the startle reflex which is stimulated by a loud sudden noise, however in this reaction the infant's elbows remain flexed and the hands are closed.

63. Answer: 3   Resource: Kendall (p. 200)
The extensor hallucis longus is innervated by the deep peroneal nerve (L4, L5, S1) and is the most common muscle used to assess the L5 myotome. The muscle acts to extend the metatarsophalangeal and interphalangeal joints of the great toe and assists in inversion of the foot and dorsiflexion of the ankle.

64. Answer: 3   Resource: Physical Therapist's Clinical
                                           Companion (p. 113)
Orientation can often be determined by asking commonly known objective questions like time, place, and year. The Mini-Mental State Examination is a short test of cognitive function often used in the screening of dementia. The maximum score on the test is 30, however a score of 24-30 is considered normal.

65. Answer: 3   Resource: Ratliffe (p. 145)
An infant would likely begin to crawl backwards at 6-7 months. The other listed options would likely occur later in the developmental process: creeps on hands and feet at 10-11 months; walks along the furniture at 8-9 months; bends over in standing to look between the legs at 12-15 months.

66. Answer: 2   Resource: Anemaet (p. 24)
Gait belts should be properly cleaned at some specified interval regardless of whether or not the gait belt is soiled with body fluid. When a gait belt is soiled with body fluid it is necessary to clean the belt before it is used again.

67. Answer: 2   Resource: Bickley (p. 326)
Hepatitis refers to inflammation of the liver. The condition is characterized by a variety of systemic signs including fever and jaundice. Transmission of hepatitis A occurs through contact with infected fecal-oral material, while hepatitis B is transmitted through contact with infected body fluids such as blood, semen or saliva.

68. Answer: 3   Resource: American Heart Association
(p. 81)

Cardiopulmonary resuscitation standards indicate that the ratio of compressions to ventilations when performing two-rescuer CPR on an adult should be 15:2. The compressions should be performed over the lower half of the sternum and should be at a depth of 1.5 - 2 inches.

69. Answer: 3   Resource: Cameron (p. 288)

Duty cycle refers to the proportion of the total treatment time that ultrasound is being generated. A 20% duty cycle would be used for nonthermal effects and would therefore not significantly increase tissue temperature.

70. Answer: 2   Resource: Minor (p. 122)

Placing a pillow under the patient's lower abdomen will cause a decrease in lumbar lordosis by placing the spine in a more flexed posture.

71. Answer: 4   Resource: Irwin (p. 342)

The examination procedure allows the therapist to compare the timing and degree of movement of each hand during quiet and deep breathing.

72. Answer: 1   Resource: Bickley (p. 599)

Depression is defined as a morbid sadness, dejection, or melancholy. Depression should be distinguished from grief, which is realistic and proportionate to a personal loss.

73. Answer: 3   Resource: Kendall (p. 282)

The trapezius is innervated by the spinal portion of cranial nerve XI and ventral ramus of C2, C3, and C4. The upper trapezius assists with the ability to approximate the acromion and occiput.

74. Answer: 2   Resource: Kendall (p. 193)

The flexor digitorum brevis acts to flex the proximal interphalangeal joints, and assists in flexion of the metatarsophalangeal joints of the second through fifth digits. The muscle is innervated by the tibial nerve.

75. Answer: 4   Resource: Best (p. 207)

Parametric tests assume that data is normally or near normally distributed and require interval or ratio level data.

76. Answer: 2   Resource: Anderson (p. 122)

Aphasia is defined as the loss of power of expression by speech, writing, or signs due to disease or injury of the brain center.

77. Answer: 2   Resource: Walter (p. 244)

Outcome assessment studies tend to compare a patient's status at the time of discharge in relation to the expected goals of treatment.

78. Answer: 4   Resource: Goodman – Differential
                                            Diagnosis (p. 185)
Lymphocytes, monocytes, and granulocytes are types of white blood cells
encountered with infection.

79. Answer: 2   Resource: Magee (p. 607)
A capsular pattern of restriction at the hip includes flexion, abduction, and medial
rotation.

80. Answer: 4   Resource: Davis (p. 101)
Listening to the patient express his/her feelings demonstrates respect for his/her
present emotional state. Actions to dismiss the patient's feelings would be
insensitive and can damage the patient-therapist relationship.

81. Answer: 3   Resource: Scott - Promoting Legal
                                            Awareness (p. 118)
The Patient Bill of Rights articulates that a patient has the right to review his/her
medical records and to have the information explained, except when restricted by
law.

82. Answer: 4   Resource: Scott – Legal Aspects (p. 83)
Spoliation refers to the intentional destruction of medical records.

83. Answer: 4   Resource: Curtis (p. 117)
Patients receiving home health services must meet the established criteria of being
"homebound." Since the patient is able to routinely go out to lunch with friends it
is clear that he does not meet the necessary criteria. Continuing to provide home
health services would be considered fraud.

84. Answer: 4   Resource: Pierson (p. 33)
Lying in a prone position results in a number of bony prominences being
susceptible to pressure injuries including the forehead, tip of the acromion,
anterior-superior iliac spine, anterior head of the humerus, patella, anterior tibia,
and dorsum of the foot.

85. Answer: 3   Resource: Cameron (p. 350)
Alternating current is defined as a continuous flow of charged particles in
alternating directions. Since alternating current is continuous there is no
interphase or interpulse interval, therefore the term interpulse interval would only
be used to describe pulsatile current.

86. Answer: 2   Resource: DePoy (p. 284)
The results section includes the data and statistical analyses. The information
may be presented in a narrative, chart, or graph form. The interpretation of the
data is not a component of the results section.

87. Answer: 1   Resource: Walter (p. 131)
A manager's role is to work with the staff to find acceptable solutions to existing problems. By asking for volunteers the manager may solve the immediate staffing problem and therefore provide the necessary time to develop an appropriate long-term solution.

88. Answer: 1   Resource: Cameron (p. 164)
The percentage of original radiating intensity maintained when the lamp is moved from 45 centimeters to 90 cm away from the target area is 25%. The percentage can be calculated using the inverse square law which states that as the distance of the source from the target increases, the intensity of radiation reaching the target changes in proportion to the inverse square of the distance.

89. Answer: 4   Resource: Norkin (p. 222)
According to the American Academy of Orthopedic Surgeons normal ankle dorsiflexion is 0-20 degrees.

90. Answer: 4   Resource: Kisner (p. 364)
Codman's pendulum exercises can be performed with the patient in prone on a plinth with the arm over the side. It is not as desirable as a standing position since it is difficult to initiate movement using the trunk in the prone position.

91. Answer: 1   Resource: Kisner (p. 718)
Massage techniques utilized on a patient with chronic venous insufficiency should be in a distal to proximal direction.

92. Answer: 2   Resource: Irwin (p. 55)
A normal sinus rhythm has an impulse that originates from the SA node and follows the normal conduction pathways during depolarization. Resting heart rates typically range from 60 to 100 beats per minute.

93. Answer: 4   Resource: Kisner (p. 326)
The self-mobilization activity produces a caudal glide that is used to increase abduction of the glenohumeral joint.

94. Answer: 1   Resource: Kisner (p. 721)
Application of local heat will place an increased demand on the lymphatic system and should therefore be avoided.

95. Answer: 2   Resource: Pauls (p. 82)
Osteoarthritis is a chronic degenerative disorder that leads to the breakdown of the articular cartilage of synovial joints. Joints most commonly affected are the weight bearing joints. Pain is typically worse with activity and morning stiffness is often present.

96. Answer: 2   Resource: Kettenbach (p. 97)
    Short-term goals are building blocks which often identify treatment priorities and
    provide a platform for the achievement of an associated long-term goal.

97. Answer: 2   Resource: Umphred (p. 755)
    The Fugl-Meyer Assessment of functional return after CVA assesses items such
    as muscle tone, state of motor recovery, synergy, movement speed, and
    prehension pattern of the limbs. The Fugl-Meyer Assessment can take in excess
    of 40 minutes to complete, however has been shown to be reliable and valid in
    patients with hemiplegia.

98. Answer: 1   Resource: O'Sullivan (p. 540)
    Medically stable patients able to tolerate intense rehabilitation for three hours per
    day are often good candidates for inpatient rehabilitation. Twenty four hour per
    day monitoring and therapies that provide assistance with mobility and activities
    of daily living are available at this type of setting.

99. Answer: 1   Resource: Hertling (p. 423)
    A grade I ligament sprain is a relatively minor injury that is often resolved in 1-3
    weeks. As a result, the patient's previous functional status should serve as an
    ideal predictor of functional status following rehabilitation.

100. Answer: 4   Resource: Magee (p. 3)
    Although a subjective report of pain is relevant information, additional
    information must be gathered prior to determining its significance.

This activity should have provided candidates with a basic understanding of the time
available to answer a selected number of questions. Candidates should, however,
recognize that taking a 100 question examination in two hours is much different than
taking the actual Physical Therapist Examination. Issues such as the environment,
concentration, and endurance, which for most candidates are not as relevant when taking
a 100 question examination, can be very relevant when candidates are subjected to the
actual examination.

The most effective way to determine if the time constraints of the Physical Therapist
Examination will affect you is to practice taking 200 question sample examinations. This
activity will not only reduce your anxiety level about the time constraints, but will also
allow you to make changes in your pace, if necessary, prior to the actual examination.

Unit Eight contains a 200 question sample examination. Additional information on
review books and computer software designed for the Physical Therapist Examination is
located at the conclusion of the text.

Content Outline

Perhaps the most valuable piece of information a candidate can utilize when preparing for the Physical Therapist Examination is the content outline. The content outline provides a detailed analysis of each of the four content areas of the Physical Therapist Examination. A thorough understanding of each of the content areas and the corresponding subtopics will streamline a candidate's preparation. Less time will be spent covering topics that are not clinically relevant to the actual examination and as a result, more time will be available for reviewing and relearning.

The chart below illustrates the four content areas of the Physical Therapist Examination and the percentage of examination items in each content area.

Physical Therapist Examination Content Outline

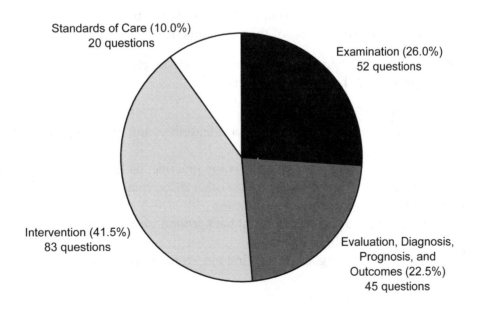

Content Outline

Federation of State Boards of Physical Therapy

Physical Therapist Examination

I. Examination
History and Systems Review

Tests and Measures Group I
1. Strength, ROM, Posture, Body Structures, Prosthetic & Orthotic Devices
2. Cognition, Nerve, Reflex and Sensory Integrity, Neurodevelopment

Tests and Measures Group II
1. Cardiovascular/pulmonary System
2. Integumentary System

II. Evaluation, Diagnosis, Prognosis, and Outcomes
Evaluation and Diagnosis
Prognosis and Outcomes

III. Intervention
Non-procedural Intervention
1. Coordination of care
2. Communication
3. Documentation
4. Patient/family/client-related instructions

Procedural Intervention
Group I: Exercise and manual therapy

Group II: Transfer and functional activities, gait training, assistive and adaptive devices, and modification of the environment

Group III: Physical agents and modalities, airway clearance techniques, wound care, promoting health and wellness

IV. Standards of Care
1. Maintaining patient autonomy, confidentiality, and obtaining informed consent
2. Recognizing scope of physical therapy practice, including limitations of the PT role that necessitate referral to other disciplines
3. Utilizing body mechanics/positioning
4. Considering the patient's cultural background, social history, home situation, and geographic barriers, etc.
5. Safety, CPR, emergency care, first aid, standard precautions

The actual number of questions in each content area of the Physical Therapist Examination can be determined based on the given percentage of examination items. The following table identifies the number of questions in each of the four content areas on the Physical Therapist Examination.

Content Areas	Number of Questions
Examination	52
Evaluation, Diagnosis, Prognosis, and Outcomes	45
Intervention	83
Standards of Care	20
	Total = 200

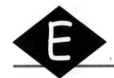

Exercise: Content Outline Analysis

The following exercise will explore the content outline in greater detail. Individual subtopics in each content area will be presented. A brief general statement regarding the subject matter in each subtopic is presented along with an outline of associated information. The information is obtained from the current content outline published by the Federation of State Boards of Physical Therapy.

Ten sample questions will be presented for candidates to answer in each subtopic. Candidates should recognize that these questions represent only a small fraction of the potential questions that could appear on the actual examination. Additional sample questions for each of the subtopics will appear in the sample examination contained in Unit Eight. Candidates should use this exercise not only to become familiar with the content outline, but also to refine their test taking skills.

Candidates will have a maximum of two hours to complete the exercise. Attempt to identify the best answer for each of the 100 questions. After completing the exercise, utilize the answer key located at the conclusion of the exercise to determine the number of questions answered correctly. Record your score for the exercise on the Performance Analysis Summary Sheet located in the Appendix.

Physical Therapist Examination
Content Outline Analysis

I.   *Examination*

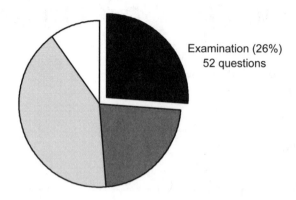

Examination (26%)
52 questions

Examination	Number of Questions
History and Systems Review	15
Tests and Measures Group I	22
Tests and Measures Group II	15
	Total = 52

History and Systems Review

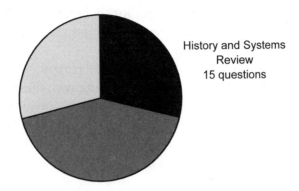

History and Systems
Review
15 questions

History

    Included are critical knowledge and skills related to obtaining past and current patient history information from medical records, and interviews with patients and others. Information includes demographics, general health status, chief complaint, medications, medical/surgical and social history, functional status/activity level, social/health habits, living environment, employment, and growth and development.

Systems Review

    Included are critical knowledge and skills related to:

- Conducting a systems review of the cardiovascular/pulmonary system
- Conducting a systems review of the integumentary system
- Conducting a systems review of the musculoskeletal system
- Conducting a systems review of the neuromuscular system

Sample Questions

1. A 46-year-old male with high blood pressure is placed on diuretics in an attempt to lower his blood pressure. What is the most serious complication of diuretic therapy?

    1. hypernatremia
    2. hypokalemia
    3. hypercalcemia
    4. hypocythemia

2. A physical therapist employed in an outpatient orthopedic clinic works with an 18-year-old female diagnosed with iliotibial band syndrome. After treating the patient for several weeks, the therapist suspects that the patient is bulimic. The most appropriate therapist action is to:

   1. discuss the situation with the patient
   2. request an immediate meeting with the patient's family
   3. schedule the patient for a dietary consultation
   4. continue to monitor the patient's behavior during scheduled therapy sessions

3. A patient with coronary artery disease is placed on antihypertensive medication in order to control severe hypertension. Which antihypertensive drug category functions by decreasing myocardial force and rate of contraction?

   1. diuretics
   2. vasodilators
   3. angiotensin-converting enzyme inhibitors
   4. calcium channel blockers

4. A physical therapist reviews laboratory testing results from a patient in the intensive care unit. An entry from the attending physician indicates that some of the laboratory values may have been skewed since the patient was dehydrated. Which finding is most likely based on the patient's hydration status?

   1. increased hematocrit
   2. decreased hematocrit
   3. increased hemoglobin
   4. decreased hemoglobin

5. A patient employed in a machine shop is referred to physical therapy with a diagnosis of carpal tunnel syndrome. The patient indicates that he is scheduled for a diagnostic test that may help to confirm the diagnosis. Which of the following electrodiagnostic tests would be the most appropriate?

   1. electroencephalography
   2. evoked potentials
   3. nerve conduction velocity
   4. electromyography

6. A patient complains of sharp pain in the abdomen that has been present for at least eight hours. Physical examination reveals tenderness in the left upper quadrant of the abdomen. Which structure is located within this region?

    1. appendix
    2. gall bladder
    3. liver
    4. spleen

7. While obtaining a patient history, it is important not to ask leading questions, which may elicit irrelevant or inaccurate information. Which of the following questions might be considered the most leading?

    1. Where is your pain located?
    2. When did the present pain arise?
    3. Which activities are particularly difficult to perform?
    4. Do you have pain in the morning?

8. A physical therapist interviews a 21-year-old football player referred to physical therapy after sustaining a grade II acromioclavicular sprain. Which of the following patient descriptions best describes the injury mechanism associated with an acromioclavicular sprain?

    1. "I was being tackled and landed directly on my shoulder."
    2. "I fell with my arm extended and another player fell on top of me."
    3. "My arm was hit with a helmet while I was throwing the ball."
    4. "My arm was stepped on while I was lying on the ground."

9. A patient diagnosed with an anterior cruciate ligament injury is examined in physical therapy. During the examination, the patient asks the physical therapist why the physician would order x-rays after already diagnosing the ligament injury. The primary purpose for ordering the radiographs would be to:

    1. confirm the physician's diagnosis
    2. check for possible meniscal involvement
    3. examine the patient's skeletal maturity
    4. rule out the possibility of a fracture

10. A self referred patient is examined in physical therapy. The physical therapist asks the patient a variety of questions in an attempt to rule out systemic involvement. Which of the following questions would provide the most direct information on the presence of a brain tumor?

1. Have you had any unusual headaches or changes in your vision?
2. Can you think of any time during the past week when you may have fallen or been injured?
3. Have you had any sudden weight loss in the last three weeks without dieting?
4. Have you noticed any change in your bowel movements or flow of urination?

Tests and Measures: Group I

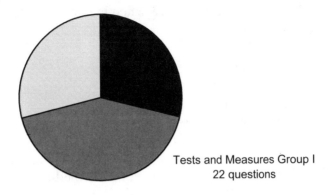

Tests and Measures Group I
22 questions

Group I:
Strength, ROM, Posture, Body Structures, Prosthetic & Orthotic Devices
    Anthropometric characteristics
    Joint integrity and mobility
    Posture
    Prosthetic devices
    Range of motion/muscle length
    Muscle performance
    Orthotic, protective & supportive devices

Cognition, Nerve, Reflex and Sensory Integrity, Neurodevelopment
    Arousal, attention and cognition
    Cranial and peripheral nerve integrity (motor and sensory)
    Motor function
    Neurodevelopment and sensory integration
    Reflex integrity
    Sensory integrity

Sample Questions

11. A physical therapist completes a manual muscle test on a patient that sustained a laceration to the anterior surface of the forearm. When performing a test on the flexor pollicis brevis, the therapist should direct the force:

    1. along the volar aspect of the proximal phalanx of the thumb
    2. along the volar aspect of the distal phalanx of the thumb
    3. along the dorsal aspect of the proximal phalanx of the thumb
    4. along the dorsal aspect of the distal phalanx of the thumb

12. A patient diagnosed with right bicipital tendonitis performs upper extremity resistance exercises using a piece of elastic tubing. What muscle is emphasized when laterally rotating the involved extremity against resistance?

    1. teres minor
    2. pectoralis major
    3. teres major
    4. subscapularis

13. A physical therapist reviews the medical record of a patient rehabilitating from a CVA. The patient exhibits paralysis and numbness on the side of the body contralateral to the vascular accident. Which descending pathway is most likely damaged based on the patient's clinical presentation?

    1. corticospinal tract
    2. vestibulospinal tract
    3. tectospinal tract
    4. rubrospinal tract

14. A physical therapist examines the cutaneous reflexes of a patient with suspected central nervous system involvement. Which of the following is the most appropriate to utilize when attempting to elicit the Babinski reflex?

    1. tuning fork
    2. index finger
    3. pointed end of a reflex hammer
    4. cotton ball

15. A physical therapist examines a 40-year-old female referred to physical therapy after spraining her ankle playing volleyball. During the examination, the patient exhibits extreme tenderness to palpation over the sinus tarsi. What ligament is most often associated with tenderness in this area?

    1. anterior talofibular
    2. calcaneofibular
    3. deltoid
    4. posterior talofibular

16. A physical therapist completes a sensory examination on a patient with incomplete T7-T8 paraplegia. The therapist examines the patient's sensation using a piece of cotton. The therapist applies the cotton in a random fashion and the patient is asked to indicate when she feels the stimulus. This method of sensory testing is used to examine:

1. kinesthesia
2. light touch
3. proprioception
4. superficial pain

17. A physical therapist determines that a patient has a one half inch leg length discrepancy. The therapist suspects the patient's leg length discrepancy may be due to tibial shortening. The most appropriate measurement to confirm the therapist's suspicions is from the:

1. anterior superior iliac spine to the medial malleolus
2. iliac crest to the lateral malleolus
3. medial knee joint line to the medial malleolus
4. lateral knee joint line to the medial malleolus

18. A physical therapist examines a patient with limited cervical range of motion. As part of the examination, the therapist attempts to screen the patient for possible vertebral artery involvement, but is unable to position the patient's head and neck in the recommended test position. The most appropriate action is to:

1. complete the vertebral artery test with the head and neck positioned in approximately 50 percent of the available cervical range of motion
2. complete the vertebral artery test as far into the available cervical range of motion as tolerated
3. avoid completing the vertebral artery test until the patient has full cervical range of motion
4. avoid all direct cervical treatment techniques until the vertebral artery test can be assessed at the limits of normal cervical range of motion

19. A physical therapist positions a patient in prone on a plinth and passively flexes her knee. As the knee flexes, the patient's hip on the same side also begins to flex. This clinical finding is most indicative of a:

1. tight iliopsoas
2. tight rectus femoris
3. tight tensor fasciae latae
4. tight hamstrings

20. A physical therapist assesses a patient's lower extremity deep tendon reflexes using a reflex hammer. Which of the following reflexes would provide the therapist with the most information on the L3-L4 neurologic level?

1. patellar reflex
2. lateral hamstrings reflex
3. posterior tibial reflex
4. Achilles reflex

Tests and Measures: Group II

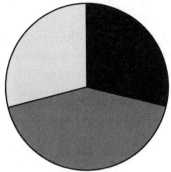

Tests and Measures Group II
15 questions

Group II:
Cardiovascular/pulmonary System
    Aerobic capacity/endurance
    Circulation (arterial, venous, lymphatic)
    Ventilation and respiration/gas exchange

Integumentary System
    Integumentary integrity

Functional Status and Community Integration
    Self-care and home management, including activities of daily living and instrumental
        activities of daily living
    Work (job/school/play), community and leisure integration or
        reintegration, including instrumental activities of daily living
    Assistive and adaptive devices
    Gait, locomotion, and balance
    Pain
    Ergonomics and body mechanics

Sample Questions

21. A physical therapist completes a primary survey on a six-month-old infant
that is lying motionless on the floor. When assessing the infant's pulse,
the most appropriate arteries to examine are the:

    1. brachial and femoral arteries
    2. carotid and pedal arteries
    3. radial and carotid arteries
    4. brachial and popliteal arteries

22. A physical therapist presents a community inservice on risk factors associated with coronary artery disease. Which of the following individuals would be at greatest risk?

1. a 45-year-old male with a cholesterol level of 260 mg/dL
2. a 39-year-old female with a cholesterol level of 180mg/dL and a family history of cardiac disease
3. a 42-year-old male with a cholesterol level of 200 mg/dL and hypertension
4. a 47-year-old female with a cholesterol level of 170 mg/dL, moderate hypotension, and a family history of cardiac disease

23. A physical therapist performs auscultation on a patient with known cardiac pathology. When attempting to assess the pulmonic valve the therapist should position the stethoscope:

1. in the second right intercostal space at the right sternal margin
2. in the second left intercostal space at the left sternal margin
3. in the fifth left intercostal space in line with the middle of the clavicle
4. in the fourth left intercostal space along the lower left sternal border

24. A patient with known cardiac involvement performs upper extremity active range of motion exercises on a tilt table. The patient's medical record indicates he is currently taking beta-blockers. Which of the following is the most appropriate subjective measure to monitor the patient's response to exercise?

1. heart rate
2. respiration rate
3. blood pressure
4. perceived exertion

25. A physical therapist assesses a patient's voice sounds as part of a respiratory examination. The therapist positions the stethoscope over the thorax and asks the patient to say "ninety nine." Which type of voice sound is assessed using this technique?

1. bronchophony
2. egophony
3. pectoriloquy
4. pneumophony

26. A physical therapist employed in a private practice observes the gait of a 68-year-old male as part of a fitness screening. Which of the following findings is most representative of the gait characteristics of an older adult compared to that of a younger adult?

    1. increased stride length
    2. increased swing phase duration
    3. decreased stride width
    4. increased stance phase duration

27. A physical therapist prepares to initiate an exercise program for a patient with diabetes mellitus. Which objective measure would be the most appropriate to examine in order to avoid significant complications from exercise?

    1. systolic blood pressure
    2. respiratory rate
    3. blood glucose values
    4. oxygen saturation rate

28. A physical therapist observes the electrocardiogram of a patient during exercise. Which of the following ECG changes would be considered abnormal during exercise?

    1. increase in amplitude of P wave
    2. shortening of PR interval
    3. ST segment depression of greater than 1 mm
    4. decrease in amplitude of T wave

29. A physical therapist reviews the medical record of a patient recently diagnosed with peripheral vascular disease. A note in the medical record indicates that the patient's ankle-brachial index (ABI) was within normal limits. The value most consistent with this measure is:

    1. .5
    2. .7
    3. 1.0
    4. 1.3

30. A 32-year-old female is admitted to the hospital after sustaining extensive burns to her trunk and right upper extremity. Which of the following burn classifications would most likely require the use of a graft?

    1. superficial burn
    2. superficial partial-thickness burn
    3. deep partial-thickness burn
    4. full-thickness burn

II. *Evaluation, Diagnosis, Prognosis, and Outcomes*

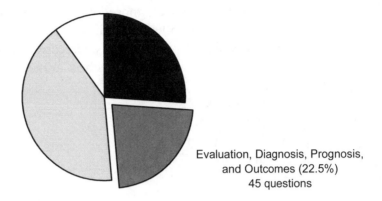

Evaluation, Diagnosis, Prognosis, and Outcomes (22.5%)
45 questions

Evaluation, Diagnosis, Prognosis, and Outcomes	Number of Questions
Evaluation and Diagnosis	23
Prognosis and Outcome	22
	Total = 45

Evaluation and Diagnosis

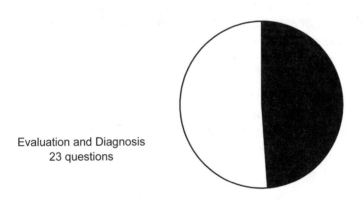

Evaluation and Diagnosis
23 questions

Identifying and prioritizing impairments
Determining the dysfunction toward which the intervention will be directed

Sample Questions

31. A 28-year-old male diagnosed with a medial meniscus injury is referred to physical therapy following arthroscopic surgery. During the examination the physical therapist identifies decreased range of motion in the involved knee. This objective finding is best termed a/an:

    1. pathology
    2. impairment
    3. functional limitation
    4. disability

32. A physical therapist examines a patient with low back pain. Diagnostic imaging reveals the patient has a mild disc protrusion at the L4-L5 level. Physical examination reveals a diminished lumbar curve and the presence of a lateral shift. The most appropriate treatment intervention is:

    1. instruct the patient in active extension exercises
    2. instruct the patient in passive extension exercises
    3. attempt to correct the lateral shift
    4. apply palliative modalities

33. A 13-year-old boy is referred to physical therapy after being diagnosed with an injury to the proximal tibial epiphysis. The boy was hit by a car and sustained a severe hyperextension force applied to the left knee. What is the most serious complication of this injury?

    1. lesion of the common peroneal nerve
    2. tear of the posterior cruciate ligament
    3. damage to the popliteal artery
    4. patellar instability

34. Documentation from an orthopedic surgeon's report indicates that a patient sustained damage to several structures that provide anterolateral stability to the knee. Which of the following structures would most likely be involved?

    1. anterior cruciate ligament, posterior oblique ligament, iliotibial band
    2. anterior cruciate ligament, medial collateral ligament, medial meniscus
    3. anterior cruciate ligament, lateral collateral ligament, iliotibial band
    4. posterior cruciate ligament, lateral collateral ligament, biceps femoris tendon

35. A physical therapist examines the gait of a 62-year-old male with peripheral neuropathy. The therapist observes that the patient's right foot has a tendency to slap the ground during the loading response. The observation can best be explained by weakness of the:

    1. iliopsoas
    2. tibialis anterior
    3. tibialis posterior
    4. gastrocnemius

36. A patient rehabilitating from a CVA is referred to physical therapy. The medical record indicates the CVA primarily involved the right hemisphere of the brain. Which of the following objective findings would be least likely when examining the patient?

    1. diminished motor control of the left side of the body
    2. impaired awareness of the right side of the body
    3. impaired spatial ability
    4. diminished awareness of disability

37. A physical therapist discusses a patient care plan with a physical therapist assistant in preparation for treatment. The physical therapist indicates that the patient has ideomotor apraxia. This condition is most consistent with:

    1. difficulty performing sequenced motor acts
    2. inability to carry out purposeful movement on command
    3. failure to recognize familiar objects
    4. inability to respond to stimuli presented contralateral to the side of a brain lesion

38. A physical therapist examines a patient who complains of occasional difficulty maintaining her balance when walking and frequent episodes of vertigo. The most likely cause of the patient's difficulty is a disorder of the:

1. visual system
2. proprioceptive system
3. auditory system
4. vestibular system

39. A physical therapist determines that a patient has diminished calf sensation and an absent Achilles reflex on the right lower extremity. Earlier the patient had communicated to the therapist that she experienced difficulty controlling her bowel movements. The neurologic level of most concern is:

1. L2
2. L4
3. L5
4. S2

40. A physical therapist receives a referral for a patient who is one week status post CVA. When observing the patient lying in bed, the therapist notes that the patient's calf and foot are edematous. The patient reports that the area is somewhat painful. The therapist should:

1. discontinue the examination and hope the patient's leg is better tomorrow
2. consider ordering compression stockings for the patient
3. continue with the examination and disregard the patient's condition
4. inform the physician of the situation and discontinue the examination

Prognosis and Outcome

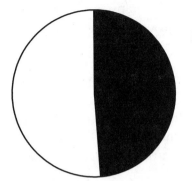

Prognosis and Outcomes
22 questions

Determining the predicted optimal level of improvement in function and the amount of time needed to reach that level

Determining the prognosis with consideration of modifying factors, e.g. age, medications, co-morbidities, cognitive status, nutrition, social support

Planning and sequencing patient interventions and progressing treatment based upon outcome

Determining outcomes

    Collecting outcome data

    Determining discharge criteria based upon patient goals and functional status

    Differentiating between discharge of patient, discontinuation of service and transfer of care and re-evaluation

    Modifying tests/measures and interventions when necessary

        Recognizing effectiveness of PT interventions

Sample Questions

41. A physical therapist reviews the medical record of a patient with Hodgkin's disease. The patient is a 45-year-old male who recently began chemotherapy treatment. What effect will chemotherapy have on the patient's ability to participate in a rehabilitation program?

    1. the patient may be susceptible to infection
    2. the patient may experience excessive fatigue
    3. the patient may demonstrate cardiac anomalies
    4. the patient may exhibit signs and symptoms of gastrointestinal distress

42. A physical therapist that recently returned from maternity leave reviews her daily patient schedule. Her first patient is a 46-year-old male that is referred to physical therapy for wound debridement. The patient's medical record indicates that he is HIV positive. The most appropriate therapist action is:

1. have support personnel complete the treatment under direct supervision
2. ask another therapist to treat the patient
3. treat the patient
4. contact the referring physician to discuss the treatment orders

43. A patient in a rehabilitation hospital returns to physical therapy after a meeting with his physiatrist. The patient indicates that during the meeting the physiatrist discussed the effect of his spinal cord injury on sexual function. Which of the following statements is typically not accurate for a male patient with complete T7 paraplegia?

1. The patient will be able to achieve an erection.
2. The patient will be able to ejaculate.
3. The patient's fertility will be diminished.
4. The patient's medications may affect his sexual function.

44. A patient diagnosed with peripheral vascular disease is examined in physical therapy. Which of the following objective findings would result in an ambulation exercise program being contraindicated?

1. decreased peripheral pulses
2. resting claudication
3. increased resting systolic blood pressure
4. decreased lower extremity strength

45. A physical therapist treats a patient rehabilitating from total hip replacement surgery. As part of the session, the therapist discusses the importance of preventing deep venous thrombosis. Which finding is the best indicator that the patient is at a reduced risk for acquiring a deep venous thrombosis?

1. ability to perform ankle pumps and muscle setting exercises
2. ability to ambulate on a frequent schedule
3. ability to achieve full hip range of motion within the allowable limits
4. ability to utilize pneumatic compression devices and elastic stockings

46. A patient recovering from a serious hamstrings strain is examined isokinetically prior to returning to track competition. Results of the examination reveal peak torque measurements of 125 ft lbs with knee extension and 78 ft lbs with knee flexion at 180 degrees per second on the involved lower extremity. What conclusion can be made regarding the patient's ability to return to athletic competition?

   1. The patient's quadriceps and hamstrings strength are appropriate for a return to athletic activities.
   2. The patient's hamstrings strength demonstrates the need for continued rehabilitation.
   3. The patient's quadriceps/hamstrings ratio is below acceptable levels for athletic activities.
   4. Not enough information is given to make an accurate determination of the patient's ability to return to athletic competition.

47. A physical therapist examines an 80-year-old female four weeks status post CVA. The therapist informs the patient that she could benefit from having physical therapy services. The patient explains that she is no longer able to drive and does not have access to any other form of transportation. The most appropriate setting for continued therapy would be:

   1. outpatient rehabilitation
   2. skilled nursing facility
   3. home health services
   4. inpatient rehabilitation

48. A patient successfully advances through a series of short-term goals, but is unable to attain the associated long-term goal. The therapist's most appropriate response is to:

   1. develop another more attainable long-term goal
   2. develop additional short-term goals which facilitate achievement of the established long-term goal
   3. contact the referring physician to discuss the patient's lack of progress
   4. discharge the patient since he is no longer making progress toward the established long-term goal

49. A patient originally referred to physical therapy for six weeks of treatment has achieved all of the established short and long-term goals in less than three weeks. The patient is completely asymptomatic and has returned to all previously performed activities of daily living. The physical therapist's most appropriate action is to:

   1. continue to treat the patient three times a week for the remaining three weeks
   2. reduce the frequency of the patient's appointments to twice a week
   3. reduce the frequency of the patient's appointments to once a week
   4. discharge the patient and send a copy of the discharge summary to the referring physician

50. A physical therapist treats a patient with C5-C6 tetraplegia. During the treatment session the patient's spouse asks a question regarding the patient's ability to transfer independently following rehabilitation. The most appropriate therapist response is to:

   1. refer the spouse to the director of rehabilitation
   2. refer the spouse to the patient's primary physician
   3. refer the spouse to the patient's primary nurse
   4. answer the spouse's question

III. Intervention

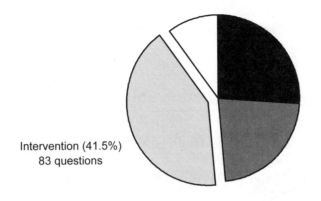

Intervention (41.5%)
83 questions

Intervention	Number of Questions
Non-procedural Intervention	14
Procedural Intervention	
Group I	27
Group II	20
Group III	22
	Total = 83

Non-procedural Intervention

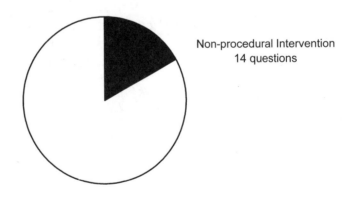

Non-procedural Intervention
14 questions

Coordination of Care, i.e., knowledge of resources and coordination with team members (PTA, RN, OT, SLHP, SW, Psychology, etc.), including appropriate referral or direction and supervision as indicated

Communication

    Educating members of other health care disciplines regarding safe, effective patient handling techniques

    Conferring with members of other healthcare disciplines about the physical therapy plan of care

    Conferring with the patient/client and family regarding plan of care, interventions, and outcomes

Documentation

    Documentation of objective, patient-centered, functional outcomes (goal statements)

    Objective documentation of examination, evaluation, diagnosis, prognosis, interventions, and outcomes

Patient/Family/Client-related Instructions

    Utilizing teaching strategies, theories, and techniques to achieve desired goals including consideration of variables that may require adjusting educational methods, e.g., learning styles, communication deficits, cultural/language style, motor learning principles

    Educating the patient/family about patient's current condition/examination findings, plan of care and expected outcomes, utilizing their feedback to modify the plan as needed

    Providing and modifying same according to the patient/family's needs

Sample Questions

51. A patient diagnosed with a T6 spinal cord injury is referred to a rehabilitation hospital for intensive therapy. The patient sustained the injury in a motor vehicle accident and has been in an acute care hospital for approximately four weeks. What is the most common type of team model utilized in a rehabilitation setting?

    1. unidisciplinary
    2. multidisciplinary
    3. interdisciplinary
    4. transdisciplinary

52. A physical therapist reviews the medical record of a patient rehabilitating from knee surgery. A recent entry in the medical record uses the term effusion. Which description most appropriately defines this term?

1. increased volume of fluid
2. increased volume of fluid within the joint capsule
3. increased volume of fluid in the soft tissue external to the joint
4. increased volume of fluid in the joint capsule and the soft tissue external to the joint

53. A physical therapist provides preoperative instructions to a 21-year-old college student scheduled for knee surgery. During the session, the patient expresses concern about his ability to balance the demands of rehabilitation and his school work. The most appropriate therapist response is:

1. ask the patient if he has considered taking a leave of absence
2. inform the patient that rehabilitation must take priority over school work
3. remind the patient about the importance of rehabilitation
4. encourage the patient to pursue university resources to assist him with the transition following surgery

54. A patient diagnosed with impingement syndrome is referred to physical therapy. During the examination the physical therapist identifies several clinical findings that indicate the possibility of a small rotator cuff tear. The therapist's most appropriate action would be to:

1. contact the referring physician to discuss the clinical findings
2. treat the patient as diagnosed on the referral
3. refer the patient back to the physician
4. discharge the patient from physical therapy

55. A physical therapist employed in an acute care hospital returns to work after a brief vacation and finds a number of items that require her immediate attention. Which of the following items should be given the highest priority?

1. a message to call a physician
2. a patient referral from two days ago
3. a laboratory test report
4. a patient record that has not been completed

56. A physical therapist examines a 43-year-old female diagnosed with a nondisplaced fracture of the humerus. During the examination the patient tells the therapist she has kept her arm in a sling sporadically, but would like the therapist's permission to stop using it. An appropriate course of action would be to:

   1. instruct the patient to wear the sling at all times
   2. instruct the patient not to use the sling because it will inhibit her range of motion
   3. use his/her best judgment based on how the referring physician usually treats humerus fractures
   4. contact the physician and ask what instructions were given to the patient

57. A physical therapist prepares a presentation on proper body mechanics for a group of 100 autoworkers. Which of the following media would be most effective to maximize learning during the presentation?

   1. lecture, handouts
   2. lecture, charts, statistics
   3. lecture, handouts, demonstration
   4. lecture, statistics

58. A physical therapist prepares an inservice on repetitive use injuries for a group of administrative assistants. As part of the presentation, the therapist develops learning objectives. Which of the following objectives would be considered in the cognitive domain?

   1. List three potential consequences of an improperly designed work station.
   2. Correctly adjust the level of a computer keyboard.
   3. Devote five minutes in the morning and afternoon for stretching exercises.
   4. Demonstrate proper posture when sitting at a desk.

59. A physical therapist receives an order to devise a home program for a nine-year-old boy diagnosed with chondromalacia patella. As the therapist starts to explain the exercise instructions, it becomes obvious that the boy is not interested. Which of the following would be the most appropriate action to improve compliance with the home exercise program?

   1. Tell the boy he can leave because it is very difficult to help someone who does not want to be helped.
   2. Continue with the instructions hoping that the boy is a better listener than he appears to be.
   3. Lecture the boy on the importance of compliance with the home program.
   4. Ask a family member to come into the room while you explain the home program.

60. A physical therapist transports a patient with a brain injury to the physical therapy gym. Each day after arriving in the gym, the patient asks the therapist, "Where am I?" Recognizing the patient has short-term memory loss, the therapist's most appropriate response should be:

   1. You know where you are.
   2. You are in the same place you were yesterday at this time.
   3. You are in the physical therapy gym for your treatment session.
   4. You are in the hospital because of your injury.

Procedural Intervention

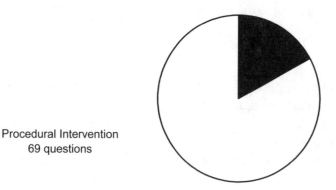

Procedural Intervention
69 questions

Procedural Intervention: Group I

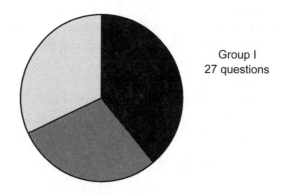

Group I
27 questions

Group I: Exercise and Manual Therapy
Exercise
    Aerobic capacity training/cardiovascular training
    Strengthening/muscular endurance
    Stretching/range of motion
    Neuromuscular re-education (including perceptual training)
    Balance/coordination
    Breathing
    Aquatic
    Postural
    Developmental

Manual therapy
    Techniques, including spinal & peripheral mobilization, manual traction
    Techniques of soft tissue mobilization

Sample Questions

61. A physical therapist administers a submaximal exercise test using a cycle ergometer. The test consists of a warm-up followed by three stages of increasing increments of work each lasting three minutes, and a cool down. During the second stage of the exercise test the therapist records the patient's heart rate as 122 beats per minute after two minutes and 134 beats per minute after three minutes. Which of the following would be the most appropriate therapist action?

    1. administer a rating of perceived exertion scale
    2. maintain the present work rate for an additional minute
    3. progress to the specified work rate for the third stage
    4. discontinue the submaximal exercise test

62. A physical therapist administers a submaximal exercise test on a patient using a cycle ergometer. The test consists of four stages, each lasting three minutes in duration at increasing exercise intensities. The exercise intensities for the stages were recorded as 50, 75, 100, and 125 watts respectively. If the therapist elects to have the patient cool down using the cycle ergometer, which exercise intensity would be the most appropriate to select?

    1. 40 watts
    2. 60 watts
    3. 80 watts
    4. 100 watts

63. A patient two weeks status post anterior cruciate ligament reconstruction using a patellar tendon autograft is examined in physical therapy. When designing the patient's rehabilitation program the physical therapist focuses on avoiding activities that place shearing stress on the reconstructed ligament. Which exercise would be the least desirable to include in the exercise program?

    1. straight leg raises in supine from 0-60 degrees of hip flexion
    2. standing hamstrings curls from 0-90 degrees of knee flexion
    3. supine short arc quadriceps exercises using a bolster
    4. gravity assisted knee extension in supine

64. A patient with patellar tracking dysfunction is examined in physical therapy. Physical examination reveals diminished vastus medialis obliquus activity. The most appropriate method to selectively train the vastus medialis obliquus is:

1. quadriceps setting exercises and biofeedback
2. full arc terminal extension with manual resistance
3. straight leg raises with leg weights
4. multiple angle isometric exercises

65. A physical therapist employed in an acute care hospital prepares to perform suctioning on a patient that is intubated. What type of protective equipment would be necessary in order for the therapist to administer suctioning?

1. nonsterile gloves
2. sterile gloves
3. sterile gloves, gown
4. sterile gloves, gown, mask

66. Which of the following goals is not realistic upon discharge from a phase I cardiac rehabilitation program for a patient status post coronary artery bypass graft?

1. ambulate 100 feet on level surfaces
2. walk up and down a flight of stairs
3. locate and recognize changes in pulse rate
4. range of motion and exercise at 6 metabolic equivalents

67. A physical therapist is treating a patient with a diagnosis of chronic arterial insufficiency. Assuming the patient does not demonstrate pain at rest, which of the following treatment techniques would be contraindicated for this patient?

1. ambulation with an assistive device
2. patient education regarding proper skin care
3. stationary cycling
4. ankle pumps with legs elevated

68. A physical therapist designs a resistive program utilizing DeLorme and Watkins isotonic training program to strengthen the hamstrings. The program will require the patient to complete three sets of 10 repetitions. If the therapist determines the patient's ten repetition maximum is eighty pounds, how much weight would the patient be instructed to use on the first set?

1. 20 lbs.
2. 40 lbs.
3. 60 lbs.
4. 80 lbs.

69. A physical therapist determines that a patient is limited in right hip range of motion in a capsular pattern. If the therapist elects to focus on increasing hip flexion, which mobilization techniques would be indicated?

1. anterior glide
2. posterior glide
3. lateral glide
4. medial glide

70. A physical therapist utilizes joint mobilization techniques for pain control and muscle relaxation at the shoulder. If the therapist begins by mobilizing the glenohumeral joint in the resting position, the limb should be positioned in:

1. 55 degrees of abduction, 30 degrees of horizontal adduction
2. 30 degrees of abduction, 10 degrees of horizontal adduction
3. 25 degrees of abduction, 5 degrees of horizontal abduction
4. 10 degrees of adduction, 5 degrees of horizontal abduction

Procedural Intervention: Group II

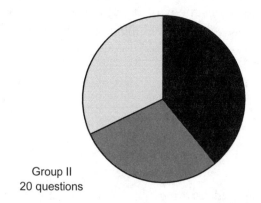

Group II
20 questions

Group II: Transfer and functional activities, gait training, assistive and adaptive devices, and modification of the environment

Transfer activities and functional activities, including safety related to transfers
    Performing transfers
    Performing functional activities

Gait training and use of gait assistive devices (normal/abnormal weight bearing status, common deviations, balance deficits, components of gait cycle)
    Performing gait-training techniques, including pre-gait activities
    Ensuring/facilitating proper weight bearing status

Prescription, application, and as appropriate, fabrication of devices, and equipment and environmental modification
    Adaptive devices
    Assistive devices
    Orthotic devices
    Prosthetic devices
    Protective devices
    Supportive devices
    Ensuring/facilitating proper weight bearing status
    Modification of environment for home/work/leisure activities

Sample Questions

71. A patient diagnosed with T5 paraplegia is discharged from a rehabilitation hospital following 16 weeks of therapy. Assuming a normal recovery, which of the following most accurately describes the status of the patient's bathroom transfers?

    1. independent with the presence of an attendant
    2. independent with adaptive devices and a sliding board
    3. independent with bathroom adaptations
    4. independent

72. A physical therapist orders a wheelchair with anti-tip tubes for a patient in preparation for discharge from a rehabilitation hospital. Which patient would most significantly benefit from this option?

    1. a patient with Guillain-Barre syndrome
    2. a patient with C5 tetraplegia
    3. a patient with hemiparesis
    4. a patient with amyotrophic lateral sclerosis

73. A patient with latissimus dorsi and lower trapezius weakness would have the most difficulty performing which of the following activities?

    1. four-point gait with Lofstrand crutches
    2. three-point gait with a straight cane
    3. swing-through gait with crutches
    4. wheelchair propulsion

74. A physical therapist examines a patient with multiple sclerosis. The patient has poor to fair strength in her legs, good arm strength, and moderate truncal ataxia. The safest means for the patient to ambulate in her home would be:

    1. with a single point cane
    2. with a walker
    3. while holding onto furniture or walls
    4. with axillary crutches

75. A physical therapist instructs a patient who is unable to perform a standing transfer how to utilize a sliding board. When using the sliding board to transfer from a wheelchair to a bed, which wheelchair option is most desirable?

1. swing away detachable legrests
2. elevating legrests
3. full length, detachable armrests
4. adjustable height armrests

76. A 16-year-old patient with a complete C5 spinal cord injury is two weeks status post injury. The patient presently tolerates only 30 degrees on the tilt table secondary to orthostatic hypotension. Which transfer would be the most appropriate to utilize when moving the patient from bed to the tilt table?

1. hydraulic lift
2. sliding transfer with draw sheet
3. two person lift
4. dependent standing pivot transfer

77. A physical therapist begins gait training with a patient who recently received an ankle-foot orthosis to assist with foot drop and sensory loss. A reddened area over the lateral malleolus persists after ambulating sixty feet. The most appropriate therapist response is to:

1. direct the patient to wear the orthosis at all times because the body will eventually get used to it
2. direct the patient to make an appointment with the orthotist and continue to wear the orthosis until that time
3. direct the patient not to wear the orthosis until modifications are made
4. direct the patient to make an appointment with the physician

78. A patient in a work hardening program is required to lift packages weighing approximately 30 pounds overhead to a conveyor belt. The patient can complete the task, but is unable to prevent excessive lumbar hyperextension while reaching for the conveyor belt. Which of the following assumptions is most accurate?

   1. additional weight should be added to the packages which will promote lumbar stability
   2. the patient should continue lifting the 30 pound packages because he will gradually become stronger
   3. the task is too easy for the patient
   4. the task is too difficult for the patient

79. A physical therapist elects to use therapeutic massage on a patient diagnosed with a hamstrings strain. The therapist can sense that the patient is unsure of what to expect during the massage. The most appropriate massage technique to initiate treatment is:

   1. effleurage
   2. petrissage
   3. tapotement
   4. vibration

80. A physical therapist instructs a patient how to rise from a chair before beginning ambulation activities with a walker. Which of the following instructions would be helpful to the patient?

   1. place both hands on the walker and pull yourself to a standing position
   2. push up on the chair with one hand and place the other hand on the edge of the walker for balance
   3. push up on the chair with both hands and reach for the walker once you are standing
   4. push up on the chair with both hands and reach for the walker while rising

Procedural Intervention: Group III

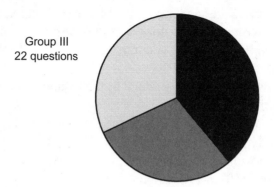

Group III
22 questions

Group III: Physical agents and modalities, airway clearance techniques, wound care, promoting health and wellness (includes some components of non-procedural intervention)

Physical agents and modalities
    Intermittent compression
    Superficial thermotherapy, e.g., hot packs, paraffin, and cryotherapy
    Ultrasound including phonophoresis
    Electrical stimulation including iontophoresis
    Biofeedback
    Mechanical modalities: traction, tilt table/standing frames, continuous passive motion
    Whirlpool/Hubbard tank

Airway clearance techniques
    Breathing strategies, e.g., coughing, huffing, and pacing
    Manual/mechanical techniques, e.g., percussion, vibration, suctioning
    Positioning

Wound care and skin integrity
    Skin status monitoring
    Patient positioning and use of adaptive/protective equipment for pressure relief
    Dressing application and removal
    Topical agent application
    Debridement technique
    Oxygen therapy

Promoting health and wellness and prevention, including instructions and intervention

Sample Questions

81. A physical therapist applies silver sulfadiazine to the dorsum of the hand of a patient with a deep partial-thickness burn. Which statement best describes the amount of the topical agent that should be applied to the wound?

    1. an amount that provides the burn with a glistening appearance
    2. an amount that makes it impossible to see through
    3. an amount that is inversely proportional to the depth of the wound
    4. an amount that is equal to one ounce for each square centimeter of the burn

82. A physical therapist administers neuromuscular electrical stimulation to the quadriceps using a bipolar electrode configuration. After observing the muscle contraction, the therapist decides to modify the treatment set up in order to increase the depth of current penetration. The most appropriate action is to:

    1. utilize carbon-rubber electrodes
    2. increase the size of the electrodes
    3. utilize additional electrodes using a bifurcated lead
    4. increase the distance between the electrodes

83. A patient with a low back injury rings a call bell and informs the physical therapist that the hot pack is too intense. Assuming the patient has had the hot pack on for three minutes, the most appropriate initial action is to:

    1. check the patient's skin
    2. add additional towel layers
    3. select another superficial heating agent
    4. document the incident in the medical record

84. A physical therapist uses electrical stimulation to treat a patient rehabilitating from a tibial plateau fracture. The therapist adjusts the parameters of the electrical stimulation to utilize a 25 percent duty cycle. If the therapist sets the on time for 10 seconds, the off time should be set for:

    1. 2.5 seconds
    2. 12.5 seconds
    3. 20 seconds
    4. 30 seconds

85. A home assessment is performed for a patient that will utilize a wheelchair. The patient's home presently does not possess a ramp and therefore is inaccessible. The distance from the ground to the front doorway is approximately three feet. In order for the patient to enter and exit the home safely and independently, the ramp should be at least:

1. 27 feet long
2. 30 feet long
3. 36 feet long
4. 45 feet long

86. A patient who is comatose due to a recent head injury receives chest physical therapy. When performing this treatment, the physical therapist should avoid placing the patient in:

1. partial sitting using the head of the bed for support
2. sidelying
3. Trendelenburg position
4. prone

87. A physical therapy department develops guidelines for electrical equipment care and service. Which of the following guidelines does not meet acceptable equipment care and service standards?

1. AC power receptacles and plugs should be hospital grade quality
2. electrical equipment should be inspected every 24-36 months
3. a file of clinical and technical information for each piece of equipment should be established
4. documentation of inspection and repair activities should be available for each device

88. A physical therapist receives a referral to instruct a patient diagnosed with peroneal tendonitis in a home exercise program. As part of the home exercise program, the therapist would like the patient to apply superficial heat to the injured area before beginning a stretching regimen. Which of the following modalities would be the most effective for the patient to incorporate into the program?

1. diathermy
2. paraffin
3. pulsed ultrasound
4. warm water bath

89. An order for chest physical therapy is received for an 82-year-old female. The patient recently underwent surgery for a hip fracture and has been taking Coumadin postoperatively. She has a history of multiple compression fractures of the thoracic vertebrae. The greatest amount of caution should be taken in the administration of:

    1. diaphragmatic breathing exercises
    2. postural drainage
    3. therapeutic percussion
    4. pursed lip breathing

90. A patient who sustained a deep laceration in the antecubital fossa is treated in physical therapy. The patient's wound has been healing poorly secondary to motion occurring at the elbow joint. Which type of dressing would be the most appropriate to facilitate wound healing?

    1. wet
    2. dry
    3. occlusive
    4. rigid

IV. Standards of Care

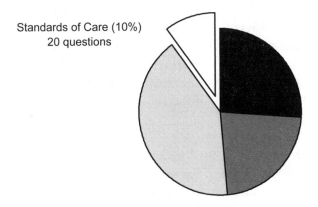

Standards of Care (10%)
20 questions

Standards of Care

Maintaining patient autonomy and obtaining consent for physical therapy and intervention

Maintaining patient confidentiality

Recognizing scope of physical therapy practice, including limitations of the PT role that necessitate referral to other disciplines

Recognizing implications of research on PT practice and modifying practice accordingly

Utilizing body mechanics/positioning
    Body mechanics (utilize, teach, reinforce, observe)
    Positioning, draping, and stabilization of patient

Considering the patient's cultural background, social history, home situation, and geographic barriers, etc.
    Safety, CPR, Emergency Care, First Aid
    Ensuring patient safety and safe application of patient care
    Performing first aid
    Performing emergency procedures
    Performing CPR

Standard precautions
    Sterile procedures
    Demonstrating appropriate sequencing of events related to universal precautions
    Demonstrating aseptic techniques
    Properly discarding soiled items
    Determining equipment to be used and assembling all materials, sterile and non-sterile

91. A physical therapist conducts a home health visit for a patient status post transtibial amputation that lives in a small two room efficiency. The therapist treats the patient for a small wound on the anterior surface of the residual limb. After completing the treatment session, the therapist would like to wash her hands. Which of the following actions would be the most inappropriate?

    1. wash hands thoroughly in the kitchen sink
    2. utilize liquid soap instead of bar soap
    3. use paper towels to turn the faucets on and off
    4. rub hands together under flowing water with soap for at least 10 seconds

92. A patient that collapsed in the physical therapy gym fails to exhibit a pulse. Upon viewing the patient's mouth it becomes obvious that the patient has dentures. The physical therapist is hesitant to remove the dentures since they seem secure, however does not want them to interfere with rescue breathing. The most appropriate action is to:

    1. leave the dentures in place
    2. loosen the dentures
    3. remove the dentures
    4. remove the dentures and utilize a mask to limit direct pressure on the patient's mouth

93. A patient who recently tested positive for hepatitis B has a one inch diameter wound on the anterior surface of her forearm. Upon inspection, the borders of the wound are slightly raised and a small amount of drainage is visible. When changing the dressing on the wound the most appropriate protective equipment to utilize would be:

    1. gloves
    2. gloves, gown
    3. gloves, gown, mask
    4. gloves, gown, mask, protective eyewear

94. A physical therapist enters a remote storage area to retrieve a piece of equipment and observes flames and smoke throughout the room. The most appropriate immediate action is:

1. attempt to extinguish the fire
2. remove patients from the physical therapy area
3. announce the code for fire over the facility's public address system
4. attempt to contain the fire to the storage room

95. A patient that has been on extended bed rest is positioned on a tilt table. After slightly elevating the head of the tilt table, the patient begins to demonstrate signs of orthostatic hypotension. The therapist's most immediate response should be to:

1. reassure the patient that her response is not unusual
2. contact the director of rehabilitation for assistance
3. document the incident in the patient's chart
4. lower the tilt table

96. A physical therapist and a physical therapist assistant employed in an acute care hospital are responsible for providing weekend therapy coverage. After examining the patient treatment list, the therapists attempt to develop an action plan. Which of the following activities would be the least appropriate for the physical therapist assistant?

1. instruct a patient in prosthetic donning and doffing
2. assist a patient with ambulation activities
3. examine a patient referred to physical therapy for instruction in a home exercise program
4. perform goniometric measurements on a patient two days status post anterior cruciate ligament reconstruction

97. A physical therapist attempts to obtain consent to participate in a formal aquatic exercise program from a patient rehabilitating from multiple lower extremity injuries sustained in a motor vehicle accident. The therapist's action is most representative of the ethical principle termed:

1. autonomy
2. beneficence
3. nonmaleficence
4. justice

98. A patient rehabilitating from a fractured humerus has completed six weeks of physical therapy and is ready to be discharged with a home exercise program. The patient is extremely pleased with his progress in therapy and gives the physical therapist a check for $50.00 as a token of his appreciation. The most appropriate therapist action is to:

1. accept the gift
2. accept the gift and donate it to charity
3. accept the gift and donate it to the department's general expense fund
4. explain to the patient that you are not permitted to accept the gift

99. A physical therapist awaiting the arrival of her next patient observes another patient ambulating independently in the parallel bars. The patient appears to lack the necessary strength and coordination required to complete the activity independently. The therapist's most appropriate response would be to:

1. inform the patient's therapist of her observations
2. assist the patient back to a chair and contact the patient's therapist
3. ask the patient if she is having difficulty or needs any assistance
4. continue to observe the patient, but do not interfere

100. Physical therapists often utilize information obtained in the clinical setting for a variety of educational purposes. Which of the following would represent an appropriate use of a medical record without patient consent?

1. informally discussing a patient's medical record with another patient
2. permitting an unauthorized person access to a patient's medical record
3. utilization of the medical record as part of a quality assurance program
4. research where anonymity is not preserved

Conclusion

Candidates should attempt to generate their own interpretation of each category and subcategory of the content outline and speculate on what type of questions could be asked. By doing this, candidates will acquire a deeper and more comprehensive understanding of the material on the Physical Therapist Examination.

Answer Key

1. Answer: 2   Resource: Ciccone (p. 309)
Diuretics function by increasing the formation and excretion of urine and as a result serve to decrease the volume of fluid in the vascular system. Sodium depletion (hyponatremia) and potassium depletion (hypokalemia) are serious side effects of diuretics.

2. Answer: 1   Resource: Standards of Practice
The patient is 18-years-old and is therefore considered to be an adult. As a result, the most appropriate physical therapist action would be to discuss the situation with the patient. It would be inappropriate to schedule a dietary consult prior to discussing the information with the patient and since the patient has been treated for "several weeks" it would be of little benefit to continue to monitor the patient.

3. Answer: 4   Resource: Ciccone (p. 318)
Calcium channel blockers selectively block calcium entry into vascular smooth muscle. This action serves to inhibit the contractile process resulting in vasodilation and decreased peripheral resistance.

4. Answer: 1   Resource: Physical Therapist's Clinical Companion (p. 141)
Hematocrit is the volume percentage of red blood cells in whole blood. Dehydration will tend to decrease the amount of plasma and therefore increase the percentage of red blood cells in a given 100 ml sample.

5. Answer: 3   Resource: Reider (p. 157)
Carpal tunnel syndrome results from repetitive compression of the median nerve where it passes through the carpal tunnel at the wrist. Nerve conduction velocity can be extremely useful in diagnosing the condition. Less formal methods to assist in identifying carpal tunnel syndrome include Phalen's test and Tinel's sign.

6. Answer: 4   Resource: Magee (p. 536)
The spleen is located in the left upper quadrant of the abdomen while the appendix, gall bladder, and liver are located on the right side of the body.

7. Answer: 4   Resource: Goodman – Differential Diagnosis (p. 38)
Leading questions may serve to bias a patient and often can generate erroneous information. Questions that are very specific have a tendency to be leading.

8. Answer: 1   Resource: Shamus (p. 400)
The injury mechanism associated with an acromioclavicular injury is a direct blow to the tip of the shoulder which serves to displace the acromion inferior to the clavicle.

9. Answer: 4   Resource: Magee (p. 52)
Although x-rays can be used to assess skeletal maturity, the primary purpose would be to rule out a fracture.

10. Answer: 1   Resource: Goodman – Differential
                                                                          Diagnosis (p. 370)
Headaches occur in 30% - 50% of patients with brain tumors. Visual changes can be caused by space occupying tumors.

11. Answer: 1   Resource: Kendall (p. 241)
The flexor pollicis brevis inserts at the base of the proximal phalanx of the thumb and acts to flex the metacarpophalangeal and carpometacarpal joints of the thumb. To resist the muscle the therapist would need to be positioned along the volar aspect of the proximal phalanx of the thumb.

12. Answer: 1   Resource: Kendall (p. 281)
The teres minor is a lateral rotator of the shoulder while the pectoralis major, teres major, and subscapularis are medial rotators of the shoulder.

13. Answer: 1   Resource: Bennett (p. 20)
The corticospinal tract carries information from the cerebral cortex to the spinal nerves. The tract's projections are primarily contralateral and have a strong influence on spinal motor neurons that innervate distal muscles.

14. Answer: 3   Resource: Paz (p. 268)
A positive Babinski reflex is normal in infants up to six months of age. The reflex is elicited by stimulating the lateral aspect of the sole of the foot with a pointed object such as the end of a reflex hammer. If the great toe extends in a person older than six months of age, it may indicate the presence of an upper motor neuron lesion.

15. Answer: 1   Resource: Hoppenfeld (p. 216)
The sinus tarsi area is located immediately anterior to the lateral malleolus. The soft tissue depression consists of a tunnel between the calcaneus and talus. The anterior talofibular ligament is often the first ligament affected by an inversion ankle injury.

16. Answer: 2   Resource: Hertling (p. 85)
Sensory testing for light touch is performed by applying the piece of cotton to selected dermatomes and asking the patient when the sensation is perceived.

17. Answer: 3   Resource: Magee (p. 629)
Measuring from the medial knee joint line to the medial malleolus allows for an
independent assessment of tibial length and also avoids any potential asymmetries
due to leg girth.

18. Answer: 2   Resource: Hertling (p. 535)
The therapist should perform the test and clear the patient's vertebral artery for
his/her available range of motion. As the patient gains additional range of motion
the test can be readministered. It is possible to observe findings such as
nystagmus and slurring of speech prior to achieving full rotation, extension, and
lateral flexion.

19. Answer: 2   Resource: Magee (p. 632)
This scenario describes Ely's test which, if positive, is indicative of tightness of
the rectus femoris (two joint hip flexor).

20. Answer: 1   Resource: Magee (p. 734)
Patellar L3-L4, lateral hamstrings S1-S2, posterior tibial L4-L5, Achilles S1-S2.

21. Answer: 1   Resource: Pierson (p. 47)
The brachial and femoral arteries are commonly used to assess an infant's pulse.
The popliteal artery can be difficult to identify due to its location.

22. Answer: 3   Resource: American College of Sports
                                                   Medicine (p. 24)
Positive risk factors for coronary artery disease include age, male gender, family
history, current cigarette smoking, hypertension, hypercholesterolemia, diabetes
mellitus, and sedentary lifestyle.

23. Answer: 2   Resource: Hillegass (p. 628)
The pulmonic valve is located between the right ventricle and the opening of the
pulmonary artery. Auscultation should be performed in the second left intercostal
space at the left sternal margin.

24. Answer: 4   Resource: Brannon (p. 136)
Heart rate and perceived exertion are the only viable measures to monitor the
patient's response to exercise, however perceived exertion is the only subjective
measure. In addition, the patient's heart rate response would be diminished due to
the effect of the beta-blockers.

25. Answer: 1   Resource: Hillegass (p. 626)
Bronchophony can be assessed by asking the patient to say "ninety-nine" while
the therapist auscultates over the entire chest. Consolidated tissue will typically
yield stronger, louder sounds while hyperinflation results in softer sounds.

26. Answer: 4   Resource: Levangie (p. 473)
    Older adults tend to spend a larger percentage of the gait cycle in the stance phase
    when compared to younger adults.   Older adults also exhibit slower walking
    speeds, longer duration of double support, and shorter step and stride lengths
    during ambulation.

27. Answer: 3   Resource: Pauls (p. 102)
    Diabetes mellitus is a disorder of carbohydrate metabolism that results from
    inadequate production or uptake of insulin. Signs and symptoms of diabetes
    mellitus include polyuria, polydipsia, rapid weight loss, polyphagia, and elevation
    of blood glucose levels. A normal blood glucose level is 80–100 mg/dl.

28. Answer: 3   Resource: Brannon (p. 226)
    ST segment depression of less than 1 mm may occur in a healthy individual
    during exercise, however changes of greater than 1 mm would be considered
    abnormal.

29. Answer: 3   Resource: O'Sullivan (p. 592)
    The ankle-brachial index (ABI) is a ratio that is calculated by dividing the lower
    extremity pressure by the upper extremity pressure. Normal values for the ABI
    are 1.0 or slightly higher. Values less than .50 are indicative of severe arterial
    disease.

30. Answer: 4   Resource: Rothstein (p. 1117)
    Full-thickness burns are characterized by complete destruction of the epidermis
    and dermis with or without damage to the subcutaneous fat layer. Since new
    tissue is only generated from the periphery of the burn site, grafts are necessary.

31. Answer: 2   Resource: Guide to Physical Therapist
                                                   Practice (p. S22)
    An impairment is defined as a loss or abnormality of physiological,
    psychological, or anatomical structure or function.

32. Answer: 3   Resource: Kisner (p. 619)
    If possible, the lateral shift should be corrected prior to any form of active and
    passive exercise.

33. Answer: 3   Resource: Salter (p. 505)
    Damage to an artery can create a life threatening emergency that requires
    immediate medical attention. The term epiphysis refers to a center for
    ossification at the end of a long bone.

34. Answer: 3   Resource: Magee (p. 695)
    The anterior cruciate ligament, lateral collateral ligament, and iliotibial band
    provide anterolateral stability to the knee.

35. Answer: 2   Resource: Kendall (p. 201)
The tibialis anterior acts to dorsiflex the ankle joint and invert the foot. Injury to
the deep peroneal nerve (L4, L5, S1) may produce dramatic weakness in
dorsiflexion and resultant foot drop.

36. Answer: 2   Resource: Umphred (p. 755)
A patient rehabilitating from a CVA with right hemisphere involvement and
resultant left hemiplegia would exhibit impaired awareness of the left side of the
body.

37. Answer: 2   Resource: O'Sullivan (p. 533)
Ideomotor apraxia refers to an inability to perform movements necessary to use
objects properly on command, although in some instances automatic movement
may occur.

38. Answer: 4   Resource: Shumway-Cook (p. 74)
Abnormalities of the vestibular system result in dizziness and impaired balance.
The vestibular system itself is stimulated by the position of the head in space and
changes in the direction of movement of the head.

39. Answer: 4   Resource: Hoppenfeld (p. 254)
The Achilles reflex is from the S1 spinal level. Sensation on the posterior calf is
from the S1-S2 level while the bowel is associated with the sacral segments of the
spinal cord (S2-S4).

40. Answer: 4   Resource: Paz (p. 376)
The patient's signs and symptoms are consistent with the presence of a deep
venous thrombosis. Referral for additional medical examination is necessary.

41. Answer: 2   Resource: Paz (p. 328)
Chemotherapy uses toxic chemicals to destroy cancerous cells in an attempt to
reduce the size of a tumor for resection or palliative care. Chemotherapy is a
systemic intervention usually administered by an intravenous line. Excessive
fatigue caused by chemotherapy can considerably limit the patient's ability to
participate in a formal exercise program.

42. Answer: 3   Resource: Pierson (p. 309)
Therapists should treat all patients as if they have a potentially transmissible or
infectious disease. Therapists have the responsibility to treat patients regardless of
their particular medical diagnosis.

43. Answer: 2   Resource: Umphred (p. 518)
A patient with complete paraplegia would likely be able to achieve a reflexogenic
erection, but would be less likely to ejaculate.

44. Answer: 2   Resource: Kisner (p. 715)
A patient with peripheral vascular disease that presents with resting claudication is not a candidate for an ambulation exercise program.

45. Answer: 2   Resource: Kisner (p. 717)
Activities requiring increased circulation through muscle pumping can significantly reduce the incidence for acquiring a deep venous thrombosis. Although ankle pumps and muscle setting exercises are commonly prescribed following surgery, higher level activities such as ambulation on a frequent schedule will be more effective to achieve the stated objective. Signs and symptoms of a deep venous thrombosis include a positive Homans' sign, swelling, redness, and warmth in the calf. Physical therapy treatment should not continue until a physician evaluates and clears the patient.

46. Answer: 4   Resource: Roy (p. 118)
The information does not include data from the uninvolved lower extremity. Other necessary information might include the ability to complete a functional progression, ROM, edema, etc.

47. Answer: 3   Resource: Anemaet (p. 34)
The patient needs additional therapy services and appears to fit the definition of homebound. Based on the surgical procedure and postoperative status, home physical therapy services are warranted.

48. Answer: 2   Resource: Kettenbach (p. 96)
The patient appears to be making progress through the established short-term goals and by developing additional, perhaps more appropriate, short-term goals it may facilitate achievement of the established long-term goal. Not enough information is given to assume the long-term goal is unrealistic particularly since the patient is making progress.

49. Answer: 4   Resource: Standards of Practice
The patient has achieved all established short and long-term goals and has returned to his previous lifestyle. There is no longer a need for physical therapy services.

50. Answer: 4   Resource: Guide for Professional
                                                      Conduct
The question asked by the spouse falls within the therapist's scope of practice and should therefore be answered directly.

51. Answer: 3   Resource: Ozer (p. 76)
An interdisciplinary team includes several different members of the rehabilitation team that function independently, however routinely report to each other through formal and informal mechanisms and may coordinate care activities. A multidisciplinary team includes several different members of the rehabilitation team, however there is less interaction between team members and communication is primarily through formal channels such as the medical record.

52. Answer: 2   Resource: Kisner (p. 222)
Effusion is defined as an increased volume of fluid within the joint capsule. Edema is defined as an increased volume of fluid in the soft tissue external to the joint.

53. Answer: 4   Resource: Standards of Practice
Physical therapists should encourage patients to utilize available resources. Many academic institutions offer assistance in the form of tutors or other academic support that can assist the patient with the transition following surgery.

54. Answer: 1   Resource: Guide for Professional
                                                   Conduct
The therapist's hypothesis necessitates contact with the referring physician, however does not indicate the need to discontinue physical therapy services.

55. Answer: 2   Resource: Scott – Health Care
                                                   Malpractice (p. 133)
Although each of the options is a viable answer, the therapist's primary responsibility is direct patient care. Failure to provide physical therapy services to a patient for this period of time in an acute care environment could pose a serious problem.

56. Answer: 4   Resource: Guide for Professional
                                                   Conduct
The physician is responsible for determining when the sling can be discontinued.

57. Answer: 3   Resource: Haggard (p. 83)
Lecture, handouts, and demonstration provide not only verbal and written information, but provide the target audience with the opportunity to observe an actual demonstration. This multitiered approach accommodates for a variety of learning styles.

58. Answer: 1   Resource: Arends (p. 47)
Domains of learning include cognitive, affective, and psychomotor. Bloom's Taxonomy of Educational Objectives identifies six levels of the cognitive domain: knowledge, comprehension, application, analysis, synthesis, and evaluation. Listing potential complications of an improperly designed work station requires knowledge and is therefore considered to be in the cognitive domain.

59. Answer: 4   Resource: Davis (p. 208)
Due to the patient's age it would be appropriate to ask a family member to come into the room. To reprimand the boy in any form may only serve to diminish compliance.

60. Answer: 3   Resource: O'Sullivan (p. 802)
A patient's question should be answered in a direct and forthcoming manner whenever possible. Frequent repetition is a component of any treatment plan for patients with short-term memory loss.

61. Answer: 2   Resource: American College of Sports
                                                   Medicine (p. 72)
Submaximal exercise testing protocols usually consist of a number of three minute stages with increasing increments of work. Heart rate should be formally measured at least two times during each stage. Heart rate should reach "steady-state" (two heart rate measurements within 6 beats per minute) before the work rate is increased.

62. Answer: 1   Resource: American College of Sports
                                                   Medicine (p. 72)
A cool down or recovery period should occur at an intensity equal to or lower than the intensity of the first stage of the exercise test protocol.

63. Answer: 3   Resource: Kisner (p. 539)
The amount of muscle force generated by short arc quadriceps exercises causes an anterior gliding force on the tibia and may place an undesirable amount of stress on the patient's reconstructed ligament given his postoperative status.

64. Answer: 1   Resource: Kisner (p. 525)
Quadriceps setting exercises and biofeedback provide an excellent opportunity for the patient to selectively train the vastus medialis obliquus (VMO). Biofeedback can offer the patient auditory or visual feedback that can assist the patient to enhance VMO activity.

65. Answer: 2   Resource: Hillegass (p. 653)
Insertion of the catheter into the patient's trachea necessitates the use of sterile gloves.

66. Answer: 4   Resource: Brannon (p. 3)
Activities in a phase I cardiac rehabilitation program typically progress up to 3 METs.

67. Answer: 4   Resource: Kisner (p. 714)
    Patients with chronic arterial insufficiency typically have diminished blood flow and resultant ischemia. Positioning with the legs elevated will serve to exacerbate the patient's symptoms.

68. Answer: 2   Resource: Kisner (p. 125)
    The first set consists of ten repetitions at 50% of the 10 repetition maximum. 10 RM = 80 pounds; 50% of 80 pounds = 40 pounds

69. Answer: 2   Resource: Kisner (p. 245)
    A posterior glide of the femur on the acetabulum is indicated to increase hip flexion and medial rotation.

70. Answer: 1   Resource: Magee (p. 207)
    The glenohumeral joint is a ball and socket joint that has three axes and three degrees of freedom. The close packed position is full abduction and lateral rotation, while the open packed or resting position is 55 degrees of abduction and 30 degrees of horizontal adduction.

71. Answer: 3   Resource: Umphred (p. 494)
    A patient with T5 paraplegia should be able to complete bathroom transfers using adaptive devices such as grab bars. The patient would possess full upper extremity innervation and limited trunk control.

72. Answer: 2   Resource: O'Sullivan (p. 907)
    Anti-tip tubes are designed to prevent a patient from tipping over while in a wheelchair during activities of daily living. A patient with C5 tetraplegia would be the most likely candidate to benefit from this option based on their expected level of function following discharge from the rehabilitation hospital.

73. Answer: 3   Resource: Minor (p. 299)
    A swing-through gait pattern with crutches requires significant upper extremity strength and scapular stability. It is often used with patients who have bilateral lower extremity weakness or paralysis.

74. Answer: 2   Resource: Minor (p. 290)
    The patient's balance and strength require the stability provided by the walker.

75. Answer: 3   Resource: Minor (p. 248)
    Detachable armrests will make it easier for the patient to correctly position the sliding board and successfully transfer from the wheelchair to the bed.

76. Answer: 2   Resource: Minor (p. 228)
A sliding transfer with draw sheet is the only transfer that will allow the patient to maintain a position of less than 30 degrees of upper body elevation.

77. Answer: 3   Resource: Clark (p. 343)
Since the patient has a sensory alteration and ambulating a distance of only sixty feet created irritation, it is advisable to avoid utilizing the orthosis until modifications are made.

78. Answer: 4   Resource: Kisner (p. 674)
The packages may be too heavy or the conveyor belt may be too high. In both cases the task is too difficult for the patient.

79. Answer: 1   Resource: De Domenico (p. 9)
Effleurage is defined as passing the hands over a large body area through gentle or deep stroking. Effleurage is often used as an initial, transitional, and/or final massage technique.

80. Answer: 3   Resource: Minor (p. 314)
Pushing up on the chair with both hands provides the most stable base to achieve a standing position. It is important not to reach for the walker while rising from the chair since the action may have a tendency to move the patient's center of gravity outside his/her base of support.

81. Answer: 2   Resource: Trofino (p. 45)
Silver sulfadiazine is a topical antimicrobial drug used for the prevention and treatment of wound sepsis in patients with partial and full-thickness burns. The topical agent is usually applied to a thickness of 1/16 – 1/8 inch (an amount that makes it impossible to see through).

82. Answer: 4   Resource: Cameron (p. 359)
The greater the distance between the electrodes the deeper the current can penetrate. When electrodes are placed in close proximity the current will flow superficially and current density will be greatest to the skin between the electrodes.

83. Answer: 1   Resource: Michlovitz (p. 116)
A physical therapist should always check the patient's skin prior to adjusting the number of towel layers utilized with a hot pack.

84. Answer: 4   Resource: Nelson (p. 29)
Duty cycle refers to the ratio of the on time to the total time (on+off time).
$10 / (10+30) = .25 (100) = 25\%$

85. Answer: 3   Resource: Rothstein (p. 24)
For each inch of vertical rise a properly constructed ramp will have 12 inches of length.

86. Answer: 3   Resource: Anderson (p. 1745)
The Trendelenburg position is an inclined position in which the body and legs are elevated in relation to the head. This position is not recommended for patients with a known or suspected head injury.

87. Answer: 2   Resource: Robinson (p. 75)
Electrical equipment should be inspected at a minimum of once every 12 months.

88. Answer: 4   Resource: Michlovitz (p. 142)
A warm water bath is the most appropriate superficial heating agent to incorporate into the home program since it is readily available and easily applied to the lower leg and foot.

89. Answer: 3   Resource: Irwin (p. 345)
Percussion is a technique that can be used to mobilize retained secretions. The technique involves direct contact over a given segment of the lung and should therefore be used with caution based on the patient's past medical history.

90. Answer: 4   Resource: Trofino (p. 43)
A rigid dressing will serve to immobilize the injured area and offer protection from outside contaminants.

91. Answer: 1   Resource: Anemaet (p. 21)
The kitchen sink is often the site for food preparation and other essential functions of daily living. As a result, it is an inappropriate site for hand washing due to the potential to spread infectious material.

92. Answer: 1   Resource: American Heart Association
                                              (p. 67)
Dentures that are not loose should not be removed during rescue breathing since they can assist the therapist to form an appropriate seal around the patient's mouth.

93. Answer: 1   Resource: Minor (p. 56)
The location and size of the wound combined with a limited amount of drainage make gloves the most appropriate form of medical asepsis when changing the dressing.

94. Answer: 3   Resource: Goold (p. 1)
A physical therapist will be much more efficient and effective in responding to an emergency with the assistance of other trained professionals. The question provides little information on the number of patients within the treatment area or the size of the health care facility, as a result the most appropriate response is to seek assistance by using the public address system. Although attempting to contain the fire through a specific action such as closing the door is very appropriate, other methods of containment such as attempting to extinguish the fire could further jeopardize the safety of the therapist and patient.

95. Answer: 4   Resource: Goodman - Pathology
                                                 (p. 296)
The most immediate response should be to eliminate the causative factor that is creating the condition, therefore the therapist should lower the tilt table.

96. Answer: 3   Resource: Guide to Physical Therapist
                                                 Practice (p. S31)
Physical therapist assistants perform procedures and related tasks that have been selected and delegated by the supervising physical therapist. It is not appropriate to delegate an examination.

97. Answer: 1   Resource: Davis (p. 61)
Autonomy is defined as independent functioning. As an ethical term it indicates freedom to decide or freedom to act.

98. Answer: 4   Resource: Guide for Professional
                                                 Conduct
The Code of Ethics states that physical therapists seek reimbursement for their services that is deserved and reasonable. Accepting a check from a patient, regardless of its use, is unacceptable.

99. Answer: 2   Resource: Guide for Professional
                                                 Conduct
The therapist has made a judgment that the patient "lacks the necessary strength and coordination required to complete the activity independently." The only method to resolve the situation and be sure the patient is unharmed is to become directly involved.

100. Answer: 3   Resource: Walter (p. 244)
Quality assurance programs are an internal process aimed at improving patient care, therefore patient consent is not necessary.

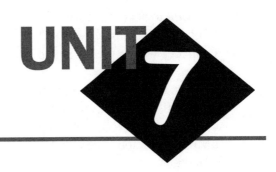

Final Preparation

As the date of the Physical Therapist Examination steadily approaches, candidates usually experience an increase in their anxiety level. Candidates often voice concerns such as: "How am I going to remember everything?" "What if I studied the wrong material?" "Did I study enough?" Unfortunately, the answer to these seemingly simple questions can be very complicated.

The good news is that candidates who have taken the time to develop a comprehensive study plan and periodically assess their progress towards meeting established goals tend to perform well on the examination. The performance of candidates who have either neglected to study or have approached their studying in a random or inefficient manner can be much more difficult to predict.

Regardless of which description best describes your preparation, when the examination is less than 48 hours away, it is simply too late to make any significant changes in your study plan. Instead, candidates need to focus on other variables they can control. This unit will offer specific suggestions for candidates to incorporate into their final preparation.

Examination Strategy

Just as you developed an individualized study plan according to your needs as a learner, you now need to consider how you can take the examination with the same considerations in mind.

If you determined you were an Active/Active or Active/Passive learner for input and processing, you may find this four and one half hour, physically passive testing environment to be particularly trying and consequently, anxiety producing. You may find yourself being distracted by every noise, vibration, and movement in the room, and may notice that your ability to concentrate has been compromised. Although it is impossible to have the same type of control over the examination site as you did over your study sessions, it is possible to make a few alterations that can be beneficial:

1. Attempt to secure a corner location. Corner locations tend to limit peripheral vision distracters.
2. Consider wearing earplugs to block out some of the unnecessary background noise.
3. Prior to beginning the examination write down question numbers 25, 50, 75, 100, 125, 150, 175 and 200 on a piece of paper and place it in a visible location. As you progress through the examination, perform a brief relaxation exercise at each of the scheduled intervals. A sample relaxation exercise is outlined in the Appendix.

If you determined you were a Passive/Active or Passive/Passive learner you may not be as challenged by the physically passive nature of the four and one half hour testing environment, but the intensity of the mental activity may produce anxiety in the form of tense muscles and a gradual lengthening of the time needed to answer each question. Here are some recommendations you may consider:

1. Attempt to secure a location where you will not be disturbed by the movements of other candidates.
2. If you concentrate better in a quiet setting, you may want to consider wearing earplugs.
3. Prior to beginning the examination write down question number 50, 100, 150, and 200 on a piece of paper and place it in a visible location. As you progress through the examination, perform the relaxation exercise at each of the scheduled intervals. A sample relaxation exercise is outlined in the Appendix.

The suggested recommendations for each learning style should be incorporated into a candidate's study plan. Candidates can attempt to incorporate the recommendations as they take the 200 question sample examination located in Unit Eight. By utilizing this information prior to the actual examination, candidates can evaluate the utility of each suggestion and construct an individualized examination strategy.

Miscellaneous Items

Scheduling the Examination

Candidates will have 60 days from the date on the Federation of State Boards of Physical Therapy "approval to test" letter to take the Physical Therapist Examination. It is important to schedule an appointment relatively early in the 60 day window in order to ensure availability at a local Prometric Testing Center. Candidates should schedule their examination at a time consistent with their optimal level of functioning. For example, if a candidate tends to be a morning person it would be prudent to schedule the examination early in the morning. Candidates with significant anxiety related to the examination may also want an early appointment in order to avoid worrying about the examination throughout the day.

Examination Site

If candidates are not familiar with the exact location of the examination site, it is often prudent to travel to the site before the actual examination date. This trip can serve two important purposes. The first is that candidates will have an accurate idea of the time necessary to travel to the site, and therefore will be able to plan accordingly the day of the examination. The second purpose is that the pre-examination visit should eliminate the possibility of getting lost and subsequently being late for the examination.

Studying

Last minute studying is strongly discouraged. Candidates should avoid studying the entire day before the examination. A 24-hour period without studying is often necessary to put the mind at ease and limit needless worry about the examination. Candidates who have prepared adequately will feel comfortable with their preparation and will go into the examination with a high level of confidence. Last minute studying will only serve to undermine this confidence.

Testing Supplies

Take time the day prior to the examination to gather the necessary supplies. Read the information from the Prometric Testing Center carefully and be sure that you have secured and packed each of the items. Failure to provide a given item, such as two forms of identification, can result in a scheduled appointment being delayed or canceled.

Dress

Plan to dress comfortably for the examination. Select an outfit the night before that can be altered depending on conditions at the examination site. Generally a blouse or shirt with a sweater can accommodate for a variety of conditions. Pants are generally the preferred choice over shorts. Light pants tend to be comfortable in warm weather and also keep the chill off in air conditioning or colder conditions. Although your clothing will not determine your examination score, it is important to be comfortable. Excessive heat or cold can serve as a distracter during the examination.

Entertainment

The night before the examination, engage in an activity that you particularly enjoy, whether it's going to your favorite restaurant, a theater performance, or spending a quiet evening at home with your significant other. By taking part in a planned activity, you will avoid focusing on the impending examination and harness any growing anxiety.

Bedtime

Make a special effort to be in bed at or before your usual time. Your mind will need to be rested and at an optimal functioning level the day of the examination. Lack of sleep or other deterrents, such as alcohol or drugs will serve to limit your performance. Use an alarm clock to make sure you are up in plenty of time on the big day.

The Big Day

As the blare of the alarm clock breaks the morning calm, your day officially begins. Since you already have performed the majority of the tasks associated with the examination, there should be little extra to do except your routine daily activities.

Special attention should be given to eating well balanced meals. Considering there will be some travel associated with getting to the examination site, and the allotted examination time is four and one half hours, it may be quite awhile until you have the opportunity to eat again.

Travel

Be sure to leave extra time when traveling to the Prometric Testing Center. Leaving additional time will allow a candidate to enter the examination site calm and collected. Arriving late or just as the examination is scheduled to begin will cause needless stress and may have a negative impact on a candidate's performance.

Show Time

Always take the available time to review the tutorial prior to beginning the examination. The fifteen minutes allotted to the tutorial does not count toward the four and one half hour time period given to take the actual examination. Be sure that you have a thorough understanding of the information conveyed in the tutorial prior to beginning the examination. If anything remains unclear, seek additional guidance from an authorized agent at the testing center. The tutorial not only reminds you of several important features of computer based testing, but also can serve as a way to limit growing test anxiety.

When taking the actual examination, read all questions carefully and consider each option with an open mind. Finish the examination only when you either have used all of the allotted time or have finished answering all of the questions. When leaving the examination take solace knowing that you did the best job possible. Take pride in the fact your preparation was both timely and effective. Resist the temptation to scrutinize and second guess yourself; it will only result in wasted energy and cannot possibly change your examination results. Typically, candidates will be notified of their results in 3-10 days by their state licensing agency.

Conclusion

We have presented a number of different strategies that, when used appropriately, can assist candidates to maximize their performance on the Physical Therapist Examination. Candidates should avoid focusing on any of the specific strategies in isolation, and instead incorporate them into a comprehensive study plan. By utilizing the information contained in the text and developing specific individual strategies, you already have taken a large step towards being successful on the Physical Therapist Examination.

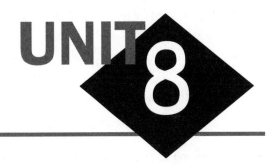

Sample Examination

As we have indicated numerous times throughout this text, candidates can obtain a great deal of valuable information by taking sample examinations. Candidates who are exposed to sample examinations have several distinct opportunities that otherwise may not be available.

1. Candidates have the opportunity to refine their test taking skills with sample questions that are similar in design and format to actual examination questions.

2. Candidates have the opportunity to assess their current level of preparation prior to the actual examination.

In this unit, candidates will have the opportunity to take a 200 question sample examination. In order to assess a candidate's performance on the sample examination, a number of indicators must be examined. Perhaps the most obvious indicator is the number of questions a candidate answers correctly. Since the Physical Therapist Examination consists of 200 scored items, the maximum number of questions a candidate can answer correctly is 200. The established criterion-referenced score for the 200 question sample examination is 150.

Unfortunately, it is not possible to identify a single number of questions that must be answered correctly in order to be successful on the actual Physical Therapist Examination. This number fluctuates based on the level of difficulty of each given examination. Candidates should use the number of questions answered correctly on the sample examination only as a general indicator of their current level of preparation.

There are a number of less obvious indicators that can offer candidates feedback as they prepare for the Physical Therapist Examination. These indicators often are best examined by answering several selected questions.

• Were you able to maintain the same level of concentration throughout the entire examination?

• Did you have adequate time to complete the examination?

- Did you effectively incorporate test taking strategies?

- Did you misinterpret or fail to identify what selected questions were asking?

- Did the questions that were answered incorrectly exhibit any similar characteristics?

- Did you make any careless mistakes?

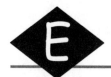

Exercise: Physical Therapist Examination

Each candidate will have a maximum of four hours to complete the 200 question examination. Candidates should attempt to take the examination in a single designated four hour period. By completing the examination in this fashion, candidates can make the sample examination more realistic, and therefore will be able to gather more accurate information on their performance.

Attempt to identify the best answer to each question. After completing the examination, utilize the answer key located at the conclusion of the exercise to determine the number of questions answered correctly. Record your score for the examination in the Performance Analysis Summary Sheet located in the Appendix. The criterion-referenced passing score for this sample examination is 150. Therefore a score of 150 or more would be a passing score and a score of less than 150 would be a failing score.

Candidate performance on the sample examination should be used only as a method to assess strengths and weaknesses and should not be utilized as a predictor of actual examination performance. Any similarity in the questions contained within the sample examination and a question on any version of the Physical Therapist Examination is purely coincidental.

Physical Therapist Examination

1. A physical therapist instructs a patient rehabilitating from a tibial plateau fracture to ascend a curb using axillary crutches. The patient is partial weight bearing and uses a three-point gait pattern when ambulating. When ascending a curb the therapist should instruct the patient to lead with the:

   1. uninvolved lower extremity
   2. involved lower extremity
   3. axillary crutches
   4. axillary crutch and uninvolved lower extremity

2. A physical therapist attempts to transfer a moderately obese patient from a wheelchair to a bed. The therapist is concerned about the size of the patient, but is unable to secure another staff member to assist with the transfer. Which type of transfer would allow the therapist to move the patient with the greatest ease?

   1. dependent standing pivot
   2. hydraulic lift
   3. sliding board
   4. assisted standing pivot

3. A physical therapist conducts a goniometric assessment of a patient's upper extremities. Which of the following values is most indicative of normal passive glenohumeral abduction?

   1. 80 degrees
   2. 120 degrees
   3. 155 degrees
   4. 180 degrees

4. A physical therapist designs a therapeutic exercise program for a patient with sway-back. The most appropriate exercise is:

   1. lower abdominal strengthening
   2. hip flexor strengthening
   3. anterior pelvic tilts
   4. low back strengthening

5. A physical therapist monitors a patient's respiration rate during exercise. Which of the following would be considered a normal response?

   1. the respiration rate declines during exercise as the intensity of exercise increases
   2. the respiration rate does not increase during exercise
   3. the rhythm of the respiration pattern becomes irregular during exercise
   4. the respiration rate decreases as the intensity of the exercise plateaus

6. A physical therapist reviews the results of a pulmonary function test. Assuming normal values, which of the following measurements would you expect to be the greatest?

   1. vital capacity
   2. tidal volume
   3. residual volume
   4. inspiratory reserve volume

7. A patient involved in a motor vehicle accident sustains an injury to the posterior cord of the brachial plexus. Which muscle would not be affected by the injury?

   1. infraspinatus
   2. subscapularis
   3. latissimus dorsi
   4. teres major

8. While treating a patient bedside, a physical therapist notices that an improperly positioned bedrail has partially occluded the tubing of an IV line. The therapist's most immediate response should be to:

   1. contact nursing
   2. contact the referring physician
   3. reposition the bedrail
   4. document the incident

9. A physical therapist designs a training program for a patient without cardiovascular pathology. The therapist calculates the patient's age predicted maximal heart rate as 175 beats per minute. Which of the following would be an acceptable target heart rate for the patient during cardiovascular exercise?

1. 93 beats per minute
2. 122 beats per minute
3. 169 beats per minute
4. 195 beats per minute

10. While preparing a sterile field for wound debridement, a physical therapist accidentally places a nonsterile object on the sterile base. The most appropriate action is to:

1. remove the nonsterile object from the sterile base and continue with treatment
2. continue with treatment, however be sure no other supplies come in contact with the nonsterile object
3. remove all of the items to be used from the sterile base and replace them with similar items that are sterile
4. discard the entire sterile field and establish a new sterile field

11. A patient rehabilitating from a fractured right humerus is examined in physical therapy. The therapist uses a goniometer to determine that the patient can actively flex his right shoulder to 173 degrees. Which of the following entries would be the most appropriate to illustrate the therapist's findings?

1. right shoulder flexion range of motion 0 - 173 degrees
2. right shoulder range of motion is within normal limits
3. right shoulder flexion active range of motion to 173 degrees
4. right shoulder active range of motion to 173 degrees

12. A physical therapist works with a patient placed in isolation. The therapist is required to wear a mask while treating the patient, but is not required to wear gloves or a gown. This type of isolation could be termed:

1. strict isolation
2. contact isolation
3. respiratory isolation
4. blood/body fluid precautions

13. A 13-year-old female diagnosed with cerebral palsy is referred to physical therapy. The patient exhibits slow, involuntary, continuous writhing movements of the upper and lower extremities. This type of motor disturbance is most representative of:

   1. spasticity
   2. ataxia
   3. hypotonia
   4. athetosis

14. A patient, who is status post CVA and demonstrates Wernicke's aphasia, is learning how to perform a sit to stand transfer. To enhance the patient's ability to learn the transfer, the physical therapist should avoid:

   1. using a mirror for visual feedback
   2. providing detailed instructions
   3. using repetition
   4. demonstrating

15. A physician refers a patient rehabilitating from a fractured femur to physical therapy for gait training. Which of the following would not be the responsibility of the physical therapist?

   1. assessing balance
   2. determining weight bearing status
   3. selecting an assistive device
   4. assessing endurance

16. A physical therapist attends an inservice that reviews regulations from the Occupational Safety and Health Administration. Which of the following regulations is not accurate?

   1. Provide proper containers for the disposal of waste and sharp items.
   2. Educate employees on the methods of transmission and the prevention of hepatitis B and HIV.
   3. Require all employees to receive the hepatitis B vaccine.
   4. Provide education and follow-up care to employees who are exposed to communicable diseases.

17. A patient status post total hip replacement is referred to physical therapy for gait training. The patient has not been weight bearing on the involved lower extremity since surgery and appears to be somewhat anxious. The most appropriate setting to begin ambulation activities is:

    1. in the parallel bars
    2. in the parallel bars with a rolling walker
    3. in the physical therapy gym with a straight cane
    4. in the physical therapy gym with a walker

18. A patient involved in a motor vehicle accident sustains a Colles' fracture and an intertrochanteric hip fracture. The patient has been cleared for toe-touch weight bearing by her physician. Which assistive device would be the most appropriate for the patient?

    1. straight cane
    2. axillary crutches
    3. rolling walker
    4. walker with a platform attachment

19. A physical therapist instructs a 55-year-old patient with significant bilateral lower extremity paresis to transfer from a wheelchair to a mat table. The patient has normal upper extremity strength and has no other known medical problems. The most appropriate transfer technique is a:

    1. dependent standing pivot
    2. sliding board transfer
    3. two person carry
    4. hydraulic lift

20. A physical therapist elects to utilize joint mobilization to increase the extensibility of the ulnohumeral joint. Which position of the ulnohumeral joint would be inappropriate for joint mobilization?

    1. 15 degrees extension, 15 degrees pronation
    2. 70 degrees flexion, 10 degrees supination
    3. 30 degrees flexion, 25 degrees supination
    4. full extension and supination

21. A physical therapist instructs a patient to make a fist. The patient can make a fist, but is unable to flex the distal phalanx of the ring finger. This clinical finding can best be explained by:

    1. a ruptured flexor carpi radialis tendon
    2. a ruptured flexor digitorum superficialis tendon
    3. a ruptured flexor digitorum profundus tendon
    4. a ruptured extensor digitorum communis tendon

22. A patient with a confirmed posterior cruciate ligament tear is able to return to full dynamic activities following rehabilitation. Which of the following does not serve as a secondary restraint to the posterior cruciate ligament?

    1. iliotibial band
    2. popliteus tendon
    3. lateral collateral ligament
    4. medial collateral ligament

23. A nine month old infant with cerebral palsy is unable to roll from prone to supine. This developmental activity typically occurs by:

    1. 3 months
    2. 5 months
    3. 7 months
    4. 9 months

24. A physical therapist working in a school system develops long-term goals as part of an Individualized Educational Plan for a child with Downs Syndrome. The most appropriate timeframe for these goals is:

    1. one month
    2. four months
    3. six months
    4. one year

25. A physical therapist administers ultrasound over a patient's anterior thigh. After one minute of treatment, the patient reports feeling a slight burning sensation under the sound head. The therapist's most appropriate action is to:

    1. explain to the patient that what she feels is not out of the ordinary when using ultrasound
    2. temporarily discontinue treatment and examine the amount of coupling agent utilized
    3. discontinue treatment and contact the referring physician
    4. continue with treatment utilizing the current parameters

26. A patient is positioned on a treatment table in prone with two pillows under her hips. This position most likely would be used to perform postural drainage techniques to the:

    1. anterior basal segment of the lower lobes
    2. lateral basal segment of the lower lobes
    3. right middle lobe
    4. superior segment of the lower lobes

27. A patient eight weeks status post myocardial infarction is involved in a phase II cardiac rehabilitation program at a local hospital. What event usually signifies the completion of a phase II program?

    1. echocardiogram
    2. initiation of a high level aerobic exercise program
    3. low level treadmill test
    4. maximal treadmill test

28. A patient being treated in an outpatient orthopedic clinic begins to demonstrate signs and symptoms of CVA, including sudden weakness of the arm and leg, unexplained dizziness, and loss of vision. Recognizing the symptoms of a CVA the physical therapist begins to administer first aid. Which of the following would not be considered appropriate first aid management?

    1. monitor the airway, breathing, and circulation
    2. remove mucus from the mouth with a piece of cloth wrapped around a finger
    3. position the patient in supine and slightly elevate the legs
    4. immediately contact medical assistance

29. Pharmacological agents eventually must be eliminated from the body to prevent an excessive accumulation of a specific drug. Where is the major site for drug excretion?

    1. gastrointestinal tract
    2. kidneys
    3. liver
    4. saliva

30. A physical therapist designs an exercise program for a woman who is pregnant. Which of the following exercises would be inappropriate?

    1. pelvic floor isometrics
    2. squatting
    3. standing push-ups
    4. bilateral straight leg raising

31. A physical therapist treats a patient with generalized upper and lower extremity weakness following a prolonged hospitalization. As part of the patient's treatment program, the therapist designs an aquatic program emphasizing upper and lower extremity range of motion. Which physical property of water allows the patient to move with greater ease?

    1. buoyancy
    2. specific gravity
    3. specific heat
    4. thermal conductivity

32. A physical therapist examines a grossly obese patient referred to physical therapy with a hip flexor strain. Which modality would have the greatest ability to elevate the temperature of fatty tissue to potentially dangerous levels?

    1. diathermy
    2. hot packs
    3. paraffin
    4. pulsed ultrasound

33. A 66-year-old female is referred to physical therapy with rheumatoid arthritis. During the initial examination the physical therapist notes increased flexion at the proximal interphalangeal joints and hyperextension at the metacarpophalangeal and distal interphalangeal joints. This deformity is most representative of:

    1. boutonniere deformity
    2. mallet finger
    3. swan neck deformity
    4. ulnar drift

34. A physical therapist discusses the importance of proper nutrition with a patient diagnosed with congestive heart failure. Which of the following substances would be most restricted in the patient's diet?

    1. cholesterol
    2. potassium
    3. sodium
    4. triglycerides

35. A physician reduces a comminuted tibia fracture using an external fixation device. Which stage of bone healing is associated with the termination of external fixation?

    1. hematoma formation
    2. cellular proliferation
    3. callus formation
    4. clinical union

36. A 62-year-old male diagnosed with ankylosing spondylitis is referred to physical therapy. The patient's referral is for instruction in a home exercise program. Which of the following exercises would you expect to be the most appropriate for the patient?

    1. partial sit-ups
    2. posterior pelvic tilts
    3. spinal extension
    4. straight leg raises

37. A patient diagnosed with piriformis syndrome is referred to physical therapy for one visit for instruction in a home exercise program. After examining the patient, the physical therapist feels the patient's rehabilitation potential is excellent, but is concerned that one visit will not be sufficient to meet the patient's needs. The most appropriate action is to:

1. schedule the patient for treatment sessions, as warranted by the results of the examination
2. explain to the patient that recent health care reforms have drastically reduced the frequency of physical therapy visits covered by third party payers
3. explain to the patient that she can continue with physical therapy beyond the initial session, but will be liable for all expenses not covered by her insurance
4. contact the referring physician and request approval for additional physical therapy visits

38. A male patient with limited shoulder range of motion explains that he has difficulty wiping himself after going to the bathroom. How much shoulder range of motion is required to successfully complete toileting activities?

1. 50 degrees horizontal abduction, 30 degrees abduction, 45 degrees medial rotation
2. 30 degrees horizontal abduction, 45 degrees adduction, 65 degrees medial rotation
3. 80 degrees horizontal abduction, 40 degrees abduction, 90 degrees medial rotation
4. 90 degrees horizontal adduction, 75 degrees abduction, 60 degrees medial rotation

39. A physical therapist completes lower extremity range of motion activities with a patient status post spinal cord injury. While performing passive range of motion, the therapist notices that the patient's urine is extremely dark and has a distinctive foul smelling odor. Which of the following is the most appropriate action?

1. verbally report the observation to the patient's physician
2. verbally report the observation to the patient's nurse
3. document and verbally report the observation to the patient's nurse
4. document and verbally report the observation to the director of rehabilitation

40. An eight-year-old female with a 25 degree scoliotic curve is fitted for a Milwaukee brace. The brace will likely be worn until:

    1. the scoliotic curve does not increase within a one year period
    2. the patient resumes all recreational and athletic activities
    3. the patient is pain free for six months
    4. spinal growth ceases

41. A patient with congestive heart failure is treated with digitalis. Which of the following side effects would not be associated with digitalis toxicity?

    1. dizziness
    2. insomnia
    3. weakness
    4. vomiting

42. A physical therapist uses a S.O.A.P. note format for all of his daily documentation. Which of the following would not be found in the assessment section of a S.O.A.P. note?

    1. short and long-term goals
    2. discussion of a patient's progress in therapy
    3. equipment needs and equipment ordered
    4. rehabilitation potential

43. A rehabilitation manager designs a system to monitor the productivity of staff physical therapists. Which piece of data would be the least beneficial to accomplish the manager's objective?

    1. number of generated timed treatment units
    2. results of patient satisfaction survey data
    3. total hours of direct patient treatment time
    4. number of regular payroll hours

44. A 52-year-old, self referred male is examined in physical therapy. The patient states that over the last three months he has experienced increasing neck stiffness and pain at night. He also communicates that within the past week he has had several episodes of dizziness. The patient has a family history of cancer and has smoked two packs of cigarettes a day for the last twenty years. The patient denies any other significant past medical history and lists the date of his last medical examination as ten years ago. The physical therapist's most appropriate action is to:

1. treat the patient conservatively and document any changes in the patient's status
2. inform the patient that he is not a candidate for physical therapy
3. refer the patient to an oncologist
4. refer the patient to his primary care physician

45. Physical therapists use a wide variety of measurement methods in their daily documentation. These measurements usually are categorized as subjective or objective methods. Which of the following measurement methods would not be considered objective?

1. duration of attention
2. goniometric measurements
3. rating on a perceived exertion scale
4. time required to perform a selected activity

46. Physical therapists often begin the interview process with a new patient by using open-ended questions. Which of the following questions would not be considered open-ended?

1. What makes your pain better?
2. Is your back more painful at night?
3. How does exercise affect your back?
4. Describe your activities in a typical day.

47. A patient is referred to physical therapy following surgery to repair a torn rotator cuff. The physician referral does not include postoperative guidelines and also does not classify the extent or size of the tear. The physical therapist's most appropriate action is to:

1. consult various medical resources that discuss physical therapy management of rotator cuff repairs
2. consult various protocols of other surgeons in the area
3. contact the referring physician and discuss the patient's care
4. discuss the patient's care with other staff members who are more experienced in treating rotator cuff repairs

48. A patient with chronic shoulder instability is scheduled to have an open Bankart procedure. As part of the surgery, the subscapularis is removed and then reattached to the anterior capsule. In order to protect the subscapularis postoperatively, which of the following shoulder motions should initially be most limited?

1. flexion
2. abduction
3. medial rotation
4. lateral rotation

49. A patient paralyzed from the waist down discusses accessibility issues with an employer in preparation for her return to work. The patient is concerned about her ability to navigate a wheelchair in certain areas of the building. What is the minimum space required to turn 180 degrees in a standard wheelchair?

1. 32 inches
2. 48 inches
3. 60 inches
4. 72 inches

50. A patient is scheduled to undergo a transtibial amputation secondary to poor healing of an ulcer on his left foot. In addition, the patient is two months status post right knee replacement due to osteoarthritis. Given the patient's past and current medical history, the physical therapist can expect which of the following tasks to be the most difficult for the patient following his amputation?

1. rolling from supine to sidelying
2. moving from sitting to supine
3. moving from sitting to standing
4. ambulating in the parallel bars

51. A physical therapist wears sterile protective clothing while treating a patient. Which area of the protective clothing would not be considered sterile even before coming in contact with a nonsterile object?

1. gloves
2. sleeves of the gown
3. front of the gown above waist level
4. front of the gown below waist level

52. A physical therapist conducts goniometric measurements on a patient in supine. When measuring elbow flexion the therapist's stabilizing force should be directed over the:

1. radioulnar joint
2. olecranon
3. distal humerus
4. proximal humerus

53. A patient two days status post transfemoral amputation demonstrates decreased strength and generalized deconditioning. Which of the following positions should be utilized when wrapping the patient's residual limb?

1. sidelying
2. standing
3. supine
4. prone

54. A patient who underwent a transtibial amputation one week ago complains of phantom sensation. Which of the following treatment options would be inappropriate?

1. tell the patient to leave the residual limb exposed to the air at all times
2. discuss the option of a temporary prosthesis with the patient's physician
3. begin residual limb wrapping
4. teach the patient to tap and massage the residual limb

55. A physical therapist transports a patient with multiple sclerosis to the gym for her treatment session. The patient is wheelchair dependent and uses a urinary catheter. When transporting the patient, the most appropriate location to secure the collection bag is:

1. in the patient's lap
2. on the patient's lower abdomen
3. on the wheelchair armrest
4. on the wheelchair cross brace beneath the seat

56. A physical therapist employed by a home health agency visits a patient status post total knee replacement. The patient was discharged from the hospital yesterday and according to the medical record had an unremarkable recovery. The physician orders include the use of a continuous passive motion machine. The most appropriate rate of motion for the patient would be:

1. 2 cycles per minute
2. 4 cycles per minute
3. 6 cycles per minute
4. 8 cycles per minute

57. A physical therapist attempts to examine the extent of ataxia in a patient's upper extremities. The preferred method to examine and document ataxia is:

1. manual muscle test
2. sensory test for light touch
3. functional assessment for rolling in bed
4. finger to nose

58. A physical therapist treats a patient with Parkinson's disease. In order to improve the patient's motor control, the therapist should incorporate which of the following techniques into the treatment session?

1. alternating isometrics
2. rhythmic initiation
3. manual resisted exercise
4. lumbar stabilization exercises in quadruped

59. A physical therapist examines a patient diagnosed with cerebellar degeneration. Which of the following signs/symptoms is not characteristic of cerebellar degeneration?

1. limb ataxia
2. nystagmus
3. dysmetria
4. hypertonia

60. A physical therapist attempts to improve neck and upper back extension in an infant with developmental delay. When passively placed in prone prop, the infant quickly falls into the prone position. The therapist plans to position the child and then use toys and play objects to get the child to look up. Which position would be the most appropriate to meet the therapist's treatment objective?

1. prone prop
2. prone over a gymnastic ball
3. prone over a wedge
4. quadruped

61. An eleven month old child with cerebral palsy attempts to maintain a quadruped position. Which reflex would interfere with this activity if it was not integrated?

1. Gallant reflex
2. symmetrical tonic neck reflex
3. plantar grasp reflex
4. positive support reflex

62. A male physical therapist is treating a 16-year-old female for a low back strain. During the treatment session the patient makes several sexually suggestive remarks. The therapist ignores the remarks, but the patient reiterates them during the next treatment session. The initial therapist action is to:

1. continue to ignore the patient's remarks
2. explain to the patient that her remarks are offensive
3. document the patient's behavior in the medical record
4. transfer the patient to another therapist's schedule

63. A physical therapist attempts to schedule a patient for an additional therapy session after completing the examination. The physician referral indicates the patient is to be seen two times a week. The therapist suggests several possible times to the patient, but the patient insists she can only come in on Wednesday at 4:30. The therapist would like to accommodate the patient, but already has two patients scheduled at that time. The most appropriate action is to:

   1. schedule the patient on Wednesday at 4:30
   2. attempt to move one of the patient's scheduled on Wednesday at 4:30 to a different time
   3. schedule the patient with another therapist on Wednesday at 4:30
   4. inform the referring physician the patient will only be seen once this week in therapy

64. A primary care physician enters a capitated agreement with a managed care corporation. The physician is paid in this type of arrangement through:

   1. a standard fee based on each patient's diagnostic related group
   2. a per member, per month fee
   3. a designated fee per patient visit
   4. a designated percentage of the actual billed charges

65. A physical therapist consults with an orthotist regarding the need for an ankle-foot orthosis for a patient status post CVA. The patient has difficulty moving from sitting to standing when wearing a prefabricated ankle-foot orthosis. The therapist indicates the patient has poor strength at the ankle, intact sensation, and does not have any edema or tonal influence. The most appropriate type of ankle-foot orthosis for the patient would incorporate:

   1. an articulation at the ankle joint
   2. tone reducing features
   3. metal uprights
   4. dorsiflexion assist spring

66. A physical therapist establishes safe exercise intensity parameters for a phase I inpatient cardiac rehabilitation program. Which parameter would be the most appropriate for the phase I program?

   1. a maximum heart rate increase of 20 beats per minute above resting
   2. a maximum heart rate increase of 30 beats per minute above resting
   3. a maximum heart rate increase of 40 beats per minute above resting
   4. a maximum heart rate increase of 50 beats per minute above resting

67. A physical therapist provides preoperative instruction for a patient scheduled for anterior cruciate ligament reconstructive surgery. During the treatment session, the patient expresses to the therapist a sincere fear of dying during surgery. The therapist's most appropriate response would be:

    1. This surgery is done many times every day.
    2. I have never had a patient die yet.
    3. Surgery can be a very frightening thought.
    4. You will be back to athletics before you know it.

68. A physical therapist identifies an entry in the medical record that indicates a patient has been experiencing premature ventricular contractions (PVCs). Which of the following does not precipitate PVCs?

    1. anxiety
    2. tobacco
    3. alcohol
    4. sodium

69. A physical therapist using an electrical stimulation device attempts to quantify several characteristics of a monophasic waveform. When measuring phase charge, the standard unit of measure is the:

    1. coulomb
    2. ampere
    3. ohm
    4. second

70. A physical therapist instructs a patient in ambulation activities using axillary crutches. What two points of control should be used when guarding the patient?

    1. the patient's thorax and hip
    2. the patient's shoulder and hip
    3. the patient's shoulder and thorax
    4. the patient's elbow and hip

71. There can be many adverse effects when patients are fit incorrectly for a wheelchair. Which of the following could result from a wheelchair with excessive seat depth?

1. decreased trunk stability
2. increased weight bearing on the ischial tuberosities
3. decreased balance
4. increased pressure in the popliteal area

72. A physical therapist assesses the functional strength of a patient's hip extensors while observing the patient move from standing to sitting. What type of contraction occurs in the hip extensors during this activity?

1. concentric
2. eccentric
3. isometric
4. isotonic

73. A rehabilitation manager develops a quality assurance program that examines the extent to which physical therapists conform to accepted professional practices. This type of quality assurance program is most concerned with:

1. structure
2. process
3. outcome
4. product

74. A patient referred to physical therapy with chronic low back pain has failed to make any progress toward meeting established goals in over three weeks of treatment. The physical therapist has employed a variety of treatment techniques, but has yet to observe any sign of subjective or objective improvement in the patient's condition. The most appropriate action would be to:

1. transfer the patient to another therapist's schedule
2. reexamine the patient and establish new goals
3. continue to modify the patient's treatment plan
4. alert the referring physician to the patient's status

75. A patient with cardiopulmonary pathology is referred to physical therapy. The physical therapist documents the following clinical signs: pallor, cyanosis, and cool skin. These clinical signs are most consistent with:

    1. cor pulmonale
    2. anemia
    3. atelectasis
    4. diaphoresis

76. A physical therapist employed by a home health care agency knocks on the door of a patient that has a scheduled therapy session. After waiting several minutes, the therapist concludes the patient is not at home. The most appropriate therapist action is:

    1. contact the patient and reschedule
    2. notify the patient's insurance provider
    3. notify the referring physician
    4. discharge the patient from physical therapy

77. A pregnant patient in her third trimester completes a series of exercises in supine. In order to prevent vena cava compression during the exercise session the therapist should:

    1. place a folded towel under the right side of the patient's pelvis
    2. place a folded towel under the left side of the patient's pelvis
    3. complete the exercises in sidelying
    4. elevate the patient's feet 12 inches

78. A physical therapist completes an upper extremity manual muscle test on a patient diagnosed with rotator cuff tendonitis. Assuming the patient has the ability to move the upper extremities against gravity, which of the following muscles would not be tested with the patient in a supine position?

    1. pronator teres
    2. pectoralis major
    3. lateral rotators of the shoulder
    4. middle trapezius

79. A physical therapist treats a child who has cerebral palsy with spastic diplegia. All of the following could be used to improve the child's ability to ambulate except:

    1. stretching and range of motion
    2. strengthening of underlying weak muscles
    3. bilateral lower extremity activities such as "bunny hopping"
    4. trunk and pelvis dissociation activities

80. A two-year-old with T10 spina bifida receives physical therapy for gait training. The preferred method to initially teach a child how to maintain standing is with the use of:

    1. bilateral HKAFOs and forearm crutches
    2. parapodium and the parallel bars
    3. bilateral KAFOs and the parallel bars
    4. bilateral AFOs and the parallel bars

81. A physical therapist instructs the parents of a premature infant on proper positioning. When placing the infant in supine the therapist should educate the parents to avoid:

    1. lower extremity extension
    2. slight neck flexion
    3. hands towards midline
    4. scapular protraction

82. A 45-year-old female with psoriasis is referred to physical therapy. The patient has several lesions on the posterior portion of the thigh extending into the popliteal fossa. The most appropriate therapeutic modality to treat the patient's condition is:

    1. iontophoresis
    2. moist heat
    3. ultrasound
    4. ultraviolet

83. A physical therapist reviews a technical manual for an electrical stimulation unit. The manual discusses several inherent electrical terms such as voltage, current, and resistance. Which of the following terms is commonly used to express current?

1. ampere
2. coulomb
3. kilohm
4. megohm

84. A patient files suit against a physical therapist claiming that she was injured as a result of a specific treatment technique. In legal proceedings, which of the following would have the most impact on what actually happened at the time of the alleged negligent act?

1. the patient's recollections
2. the therapist's recollections
3. the referring physician's initial examination
4. the physical therapist's daily documentation

85. A physical therapist instructs a patient to ascend stairs using axillary crutches. Which of the following statements most accurately reflects proper guarding technique?

1. the therapist is positioned posterior and lateral on the affected side behind the patient
2. the therapist is positioned anterior and lateral on the affected side in front of the patient
3. the therapist is positioned posterior and lateral on the nonaffected side behind the patient
4. the therapist is positioned anterior and lateral on the nonaffected side behind the patient

86. A physical therapist prepares a patient education program for an individual with chronic venous insufficiency. Which of the following would not be appropriate to include in the patient education program?

1. wear shoes that accommodate to the size and shape of your feet
2. observe your skin daily for breakdown
3. wear your compression stockings only at night
4. keep your feet elevated as much as possible throughout the day

87. A 72-year-old female six weeks status post CVA is scheduled for discharge from an acute rehabilitation hospital in one week. At the present time the patient is unable to ambulate and requires maximal assistance to complete most transfers. Prior to her CVA the patient lived alone in an apartment on the first floor. The most appropriate discharge plan would be:

1. home without support services
2. home with a home health aide during the day
3. home with physical therapy three times per week
4. a nursing facility

88. A physical therapist instructs a patient in breathing exercises to improve ventilation and oxygenation. The therapist's treatment objective emphasizes the expansion of a selected area of the chest wall during inspiration. The most appropriate breathing exercise to achieve the desired outcome is:

1. deep breathing
2. diaphragmatic breathing
3. segmental breathing
4. abdominal breathing

89. A graded exercise test is performed on a patient with pulmonary disease. During the test the physical therapist identifies that the patient's systolic blood pressure has decreased by 20 mm Hg. The most appropriate action is to:

1. continue the graded exercise test
2. discontinue the graded exercise test
3. assess the patient's respiration rate
4. assess the patient's forced expiratory volume in one second

90. A physical therapist prepares to perform manual vibration as a means of airway clearance with a patient diagnosed with chronic obstructive pulmonary disease. When performing vibration the most appropriate form of manual contact over the affected lung segment is:

1. contact with a cupped hand
2. contact with the entire palmar surface of the hand
3. contact with the ulnar border of the hand
4. contact with the distal phalanx of the middle finger

The following information should be used to answer questions 91 and 92:

A physical therapist examines a 72-year-old female recently admitted to an acute care hospital following complications from elective surgery. The patient is moderately obese and has a lengthy medical history including diabetes mellitus. Prior to beginning the treatment session the therapist reviews the patient's medical record.

91. Which measure would provide the most valuable information on the impact of the patient's diabetes on her ability to participate in an exercise program?

    1. arterial blood gas analysis
    2. blood glucose level
    3. oxygen saturation rate
    4. blood pressure

92. The following day the therapist notices that the patient's breath has a very distinctive fruity odor. The patient complains of feeling nauseous and very weak. An entry in the medical record indicates that the patient had diarrhea during the night. This type of scenario is most consistent with:

    1. respiratory acidosis
    2. respiratory alkalosis
    3. metabolic acidosis
    4. metabolic alkalosis

93. A physical therapist determines that a patient rehabilitating from ankle surgery has consistent difficulty with functional activities that emphasize the frontal plane. Which of the following would be the most difficult for the patient?

    1. anterior lunge
    2. 6 inch lateral step down
    3. 6 inch posterior step up
    4. 8 inch posterior step down

94. A patient rehabilitating from a radial head fracture is examined in physical therapy. During the examination, the physical therapist notes that the patient appears to have an elbow flexion contracture. Which of the following would not serve as an appropriate active exercise technique to increase range of motion?

    1. contract-relax
    2. hold-relax
    3. maintained pressure
    4. rhythmic stabilization

95. A physical therapist monitors a patient's pulse after ambulation activities. The therapist notes that at times the rhythm of the pulse is irregular. When assessing the patient's pulse rate, the therapist should measure the patients pulse for:

1. 10 seconds
2. 15 seconds
3. 30 seconds
4. 60 seconds

96. A physical therapist adjusts the height of the parallel bars in preparation for ambulation activities. When at the appropriate height, the parallel bars should provide:

1. 5 - 15 degrees of elbow flexion
2. 15 - 25 degrees of elbow flexion
3. 30 - 40 degrees of elbow flexion
4. 35 - 45 degrees of elbow flexion

97. A physical therapist positions a patient in sitting prior to administering bronchial drainage. Which lung segment would require the patient to be in this position?

1. anterior basal segments of the lower lobes
2. posterior apical segments of the upper lobes
3. posterior basal segments of the lower lobes
4. right middle lobe

98. When examining a patient for a wheelchair, a physical therapist determines that the patient's hip width in sitting and the measurement from the back of the buttocks to the popliteal space are each 16 inches. Given these measurements, which of the following wheelchair sizes would best fit this patient?

1. seat width 16 inches, seat depth 14 inches
2. seat width 18 inches, seat depth 18 inches
3. seat width 16 inches, seat depth 18 inches
4. seat width 18 inches, seat depth 14 inches

99. A patient recently admitted to the hospital with an acute illness is referred to physical therapy. During a scheduled treatment session the patient asks what effect anemia will have on his ability to complete a formal exercise program. The most appropriate therapist response is:

   1. you may feel as though your muscles are weak
   2. you may experience frequent nausea
   3. your aerobic capacity may be reduced
   4. you may have a tendency to become fatigued

100. When performing range of motion exercises with a patient who sustained a head injury, a physical therapist notes that the patient lacks full elbow extension and classifies the end-feel as hard. The most likely cause is:

   1. heterotopic ossification
   2. spasticity of the biceps
   3. anterior capsular tightness
   4. triceps weakness

101. A patient rehabilitating from injuries sustained in a motor vehicle accident is referred to physical therapy for gait training with an appropriate assistive device. The physical therapist attempts to instruct the patient using axillary crutches, but feels the assistive device does not offer the patient enough stability or support. Which of the following assistive devices would be the most appropriate for the patient?

   1. walker
   2. cane
   3. Lofstrand crutches
   4. parallel bars

102. A physical therapist develops a problem list after examining a patient with a transtibial amputation. Which of the following would be the most appropriate entry in the patient problem list?

   1. donning and doffing prosthesis requires verbal cues
   2. donning and doffing prosthesis requires verbal cues and minimal assist of one
   3. dependence with donning and doffing prosthesis
   4. independent donning and doffing prosthesis in one week

103. The director of rehabilitation in an orthopedic private practice prepares a list of interview questions for applicants applying for a vacant position. Which of the following would be an acceptable interview question?

    1. Are you in good health?
    2. How much weight can you lift?
    3. Have you held a position like this in the past?
    4. Have you ever filed a workers' compensation claim?

104. A 42-year-old female who is unable to satisfactorily control the retention and release of urine uses a catheter. Which type of urinary catheter would not be appropriate for the patient?

    1. indwelling urinary catheter
    2. external urinary catheter
    3. Foley catheter
    4. suprapubic catheter

105. A patient ambulating with an IV in place should be instructed to grasp the IV pole at what level?

    1. a level where the infusion site is above heart level
    2. a level where the infusion site is at heart level
    3. a level where the infusion site is below heart level
    4. a patient with an IV in place should not participate in ambulation activities

106. A physical therapist monitors a 6 foot 3 inch, 275 pound, male's blood pressure using the brachial artery. Which of the following is most important when selecting an appropriate size blood pressure cuff?

    1. patient age
    2. percent body fat
    3. somatotype
    4. extremity circumference

107. A physical therapist attends an inservice on documentation as part of a quality assurance initiative. Which of the following suggestions to improve documentation would not be useful?

1. avoid empty or open lines between entries in the medical record
2. make sure all entries in the medical record are typewritten
3. use abbreviations that have been standardized or accepted by a specific facility or the profession
4. co-sign the entries of other medical personnel when necessary according to state and facility requirements

108. A patient informs a physical therapist that he has to use the bathroom immediately after being transported outside the hospital to practice car transfers. The physical therapist's most appropriate response to meet the patient's physical need is to:

1. ask the patient if it is an emergency
2. complete the transfer training as quickly as possible and allow the patient to use the bathroom
3. transport the patient back into the hospital to use the bathroom
4. instruct the patient that in the future he should use the bathroom before beginning physical therapy

109. A physical therapist examines a patient four days status post total hip replacement. The patient's medical record indicates the surgeon utilized an anterolateral surgical approach. Which of the following motions would be the most important to restrict during the initial phase of rehabilitation?

1. knee extension
2. knee flexion
3. hip lateral rotation
4. hip medial rotation

110. A physical therapist monitors a patient's pulse rate using the radial artery. Which of the following general statements regarding pulse rate is not accurate?

1. pulse rate is increased with physical exertion
2. pulse rate is decreased during relaxation or sleep
3. pulse rate is decreased with anxiety or stress
4. pulse rate is higher in children than adults

111. A patient informs a physical therapist how frustrated she feels after being examined by her physician. The patient explains that she becomes so nervous, she cannot ask any questions during scheduled office visits. The therapist's most appropriate response is to:

1. offer to go with the patient to her next scheduled physician visit
2. offer to call the physician and ask any relevant questions
3. suggest that the patient write down questions for the physician and bring them with her to the next scheduled visit
4. tell the patient it is a very normal response to be nervous in the presence of a physician

112. A physical therapist observes an electrocardiogram of a patient on beta blockers. Which of the following ECG changes could be facilitated by beta blockers?

1. bradycardia
2. tachycardia
3. increased AV conduction time
4. ST segment sagging

113. A physical therapist instructs a patient with acute Achilles tendonitis in a home exercise program. As part of the program, the therapist attempts to reduce the inflammation in the involved region. Which of the following modalities would be the most beneficial to achieve the therapist's goal?

1. continuous ultrasound
2. pulsed ultrasound
3. ice massage
4. whirlpool

114. An athlete is forced to contemplate knee surgery after spraining the anterior cruciate ligament while playing soccer. Which situation would provide the most direct support for an anterior cruciate ligament reconstruction?

1. grade III ACL and grade I PCL injury
2. grade III ACL sprain with a lateral meniscus tear
3. grade II ACL sprain with a medial meniscus tear
4. functional instability

115. A physical therapist asks a patient who has been inconsistent with his attendance in physical therapy, why he is having difficulty keeping scheduled appointments. The patient responds that it is difficult to understand the scheduling card that lists the appointments. The therapist's most appropriate action would be to:

    1. contact the referring physician to discuss the patient's poor attendance in therapy
    2. make sure the patient is given a scheduling card at the conclusion of each session
    3. write down the patient's appointments on a piece of paper in a manner that the patient can understand
    4. discharge the patient from physical therapy

116. A patient status post coronary artery bypass graft exercises in a phase I cardiac rehabilitation program. During exercise the patient's pulse rate is measured as 125 beats/minute and her respiration rate is 32 breaths/minute. Based on the patient's vital signs, the physical therapist's most immediate response should be to:

    1. stop the exercise session and continue to monitor the patient's vital signs
    2. continue with the exercise session and continue to monitor the patient's vital signs
    3. notify the referring physician of the patient's vital signs
    4. document the patient's response to exercise in the medical record

117. A physical therapist reviews the medical chart of a patient diagnosed with a fracture of the lower thoracic spine. The chart indicates the patient has worn an anterior control thoracolumbar-sacral-orthosis (TLSO) for eight weeks. What is the primary purpose of the anterior control TLSO?

    1. prevent thoracic flexion
    2. prevent thoracic extension
    3. prevent lumbar flexion
    4. prevent lumbar extension

118. Which of the following can be used to examine and objectively document motor return in a patient with hemiplegia?

    1. Tinetti Balance and Gait Assessment Scale
    2. Somatosensory Organization Test
    3. Functional Independence Measure
    4. Fugl-Meyer Assessment of Motor Performance

119. A physical therapist palpates proximally along the lateral border of the fifth metatarsal of a patient's foot. Which bone would be palpable as the therapist continues to palpate proximally along the lateral border of the foot?

1. cuboid
2. second cuneiform
3. third cuneiform
4. navicular

120. A physical therapist establishes the following short-term goal for a patient rehabilitating from total knee replacement surgery: Patient will ambulate with walker 50% weight bearing and moderate assist of 1 for 20 feet within one week. Three days later, the patient successfully achieves the established goal. Which of the following would be the most appropriate revision of the short-term goal?

1. ambulate with walker 25% weight bearing and moderate assist of 1 for 30 feet within one week
2. ambulate with walker 50% weight bearing and moderate assist of 2 for 30 feet within one week
3. ambulate with walker 50% weight bearing and minimal assist of 1 for 30 feet within one week
4. ambulate with the walker 25% weight bearing and minimal assist of 1 for 10 feet within one week

121. A physician orders a nasogastric tube for a patient on an acute rehabilitation unit. Which of the following does not accurately describe a potential use of the nasogastric tube?

1. administer medications directly into the gastrointestinal tract
2. obtain gastric specimens
3. remove fluid or gas from the stomach
4. obtain venous blood samples from the stomach

122. A physical therapist verbally warns a patient about the risks of using an assistive device incorrectly. Which of the following assistive devices would result in the axillary vessels and nerves being most susceptible to injury?

1. walker
2. axillary crutches
3. Lofstrand crutches
4. parallel bars

123. A physical therapist conducts a goniometric assessment of the wrist and hand. When determining the available range of motion for thumb flexion, the therapist should align the axis of the goniometer over the:

1. dorsal aspect of the first interphalangeal joint
2. palmar aspect of the first carpometacarpal joint
3. midway between the dorsal aspect of the first and second carpometacarpal joints
4. midway between the palmar aspect of the first and second carpometacarpal joints

124. A physical therapist examines a patient status post amputation. Which amputation level would be most susceptible to a hip flexion contracture?

1. transfemoral
2. knee disarticulate
3. long transtibial
4. short transtibial

125. A physical therapist examines a patient diagnosed with post-polio syndrome. Which of the following areas is the least likely to be affected based on the patient's diagnosis?

1. strength
2. sensation
3. endurance
4. functional mobility

126. When observing a patient ambulating, a physical therapist notes that the patient's gait has the following characteristics: narrow base of support, short bilateral step length, and decreased trunk rotation. This gait pattern is often observed in patients with a diagnosis of:

1. CVA
2. Parkinson's disease
3. post-polio syndrome
4. multiple sclerosis

127. A physical therapist attempts to assess a patient's fine motor coordination following wrist surgery. Which of the following tasks would require the greatest fine motor coordination?

1. stacking large blocks
2. assembling small pins, collars, and washers
3. turning cards
4. picking up large heavy objects

128. A physical therapist records a patient's vital signs prior to initiating treatment. Which individual would you expect to have the lowest systolic blood pressure?

1. 10-year-old male
2. 30-year-old female
3. 50-year-old male
4. 70-year-old female

129. A physical therapist designs a cardiovascular training program for a 29-year-old male rehabilitating from a lower extremity injury. The patient has no known cardiovascular pathology and has been cleared for exercise by his physician. The patient's age predicted maximum heart rate during exercise should be calculated as:

1. 170 beats per minute
2. 180 beats per minute
3. 191 beats per minute
4. 201 beats per minute

130. A physical therapist prepares to delegate an activity to a physical therapy aide. Which of the following activities would not be appropriate for the aide to perform?

1. cleaning and maintaining exercise equipment
2. transporting patients
3. preparing a treatment area
4. implementing an exercise program

131. A physical therapist prepares to complete an assisted standing pivot transfer with a patient that requires moderate assistance. In order to increase a patient's independence with the transfer, which of the following instructions would be the most appropriate?

1. I want you to help me perform the transfer.
2. Try to utilize your own strength to complete the transfer.
3. Only grab onto me if it is absolutely necessary.
4. Use the power in your legs to assist you during the transfer.

132. A physical therapist assesses the ligamentous integrity of a patient's knee by completing a series of special tests. The most accurate way to determine if the patient's ligamentous integrity is compromised is to:

1. compare the millimeters of ligamentous laxity to established norms
2. instruct the referring physician to order radiographs
3. compare the ligamentous laxity in the involved knee to the uninvolved knee
4. compare the ligamentous laxity to other patients in the clinic without knee pathology

133. A physical therapist examines a 48-year-old male with degenerative joint disease. The referring physician indicates that the patient should be seen in physical therapy three times per week. During the examination the patient indicates that the car ride to therapy takes approximately 50 minutes and that child care duties make frequent physical therapy visits impossible. The therapist's most appropriate action is to:

1. reduce the number of weekly visits and notify the referring physician
2. transfer the patient to another therapist's schedule
3. ask the patient to discuss the matter with his physician
4. treat the patient three times per week

134. A physical therapist instructs a patient with a lower extremity amputation to wrap her residual limb. Which of the following would be the least acceptable method of securing the bandage?

1. clips
2. safety pins
3. tape
4. velcro

135. A patient uses transcutaneous electrical neuromuscular stimulation for pain modulation. Which set of parameters best describes conventional TENS?

    1. 50-100 pps, short phase duration, low intensity
    2. 100-150 pps, short phase duration, high intensity
    3. 150-200 pps, long phase duration, low intensity
    4. 200-250 pps, short phase duration, low intensity

136. A physical therapist observes a patient's skin shortly after applying moist heat to the low back. The therapist identifies several signs of heat intolerance including uneven blotching and a surface rash. The most appropriate action is to:

    1. continue with the present treatment
    2. select an alternate superficial heating agent
    3. limit moist heat exposure to five minutes
    4. discontinue the moist heat and document the findings

137. A physical therapist works with a patient rehabilitating from a traumatic brain injury on a mat program. The program emphasizes various developmental positions to prepare the patient for ambulation activities. Which developmental position would be the most demanding?

    1. hooklying
    2. quadruped
    3. kneeling
    4. modified plantigrade

138. A severely disabled patient is referred to physical therapy for gait training. The patient exhibits good balance and coordination and has normal upper extremity strength. The patient currently is using a wheelchair for the majority of her transportation and occasionally uses a swing-to gait pattern with Lofstrand crutches. The patient reports being frustrated by the lack of speed using the swing-to gait and would like to learn an alternate gait pattern. What gait pattern would be the most appropriate for the patient?

    1. two-point
    2. three-point
    3. four-point
    4. swing-through

139. A physical therapist prepares a patient status post CVA with global aphasia for discharge from a rehabilitation hospital. The patient will be returning home with her husband and daughter. The most appropriate form of education to facilitate a safe discharge is to:

1. perform hands on training sessions with the patient and family members
2. videotape the patient performing transfers and ADLs
3. provide written instructions on all ADLs and functional tasks
4. meet with family members to discuss the patient's present status and abilities

140. A physical therapist treats a 36-year-old male status post knee surgery. The therapist performs goniometric measurements to quantify the extent of the patient's extension lag. Which of the following would not provide a plausible rationale for the extension lag?

1. muscle weakness
2. bony obstruction
3. inhibition by pain
4. patient apprehension

141. A patient successfully completes ten anterior lunges. The physical therapist would like to modify the activity to maximally challenge the patient in the sagittal plane. Which of the following modifications would be the most appropriate?

1. anterior lunge with concurrent bilateral elbow flexion to 45 degrees with five pound weights
2. anterior lunge with concurrent bilateral shoulder flexion to 90 degrees with five pound weights
3. anterior lunge with concurrent unilateral shoulder flexion to 90 degrees with a five pound weight
4. anterior lunge with concurrent bilateral shoulder abduction to 45 degrees with five pound weights

142. A physical therapist teaches a patient positioned in supine to posteriorly rotate her pelvis. The patient has full active and passive range of motion in the upper extremities, but is unable to achieve full shoulder flexion while maintaining the posterior pelvic tilt. Which of the following could best explain these findings?

1. capsular tightness
2. latissimus dorsi tightness
3. pectoralis minor tightness
4. quadratus lumborum tightness

143. A clinical instructor asks a student to complete three selected joint mobilization techniques on a patient diagnosed with adhesive capsulitis. Which learning domain is emphasized with the desired task?

    1. cognitive
    2. psychomotor
    3. affective
    4. psychosocial

144. A patient sustains a deep laceration on the right thigh after falling into a modality cart. The laceration causes immediate and excessive bleeding. The physical therapist should first:

    1. apply direct pressure over the laceration
    2. examine the lower extremity
    3. put on gloves
    4. contact the chief physical therapist

145. As part of an examination, a physical therapist develops long-term goals for a patient who has complete tetraplegia at the C5 level. All of the following are appropriate long-term goals for this patient except:

    1. complete lower extremity self range of motion in bed independently
    2. eat independently with adaptive equipment
    3. propel a manual wheelchair 15 feet on level surfaces independently
    4. direct a caretaker to perform a car transfer

146. A patient with paraplegia is interested in learning how to perform a wheelie to assist with community mobility. The patient is independent with basic wheelchair propulsion. When instructing the patient to perform a wheelie, the physical therapist first should teach the patient to:

    1. make small adjustments (forward and backward) after being placed in the wheelie position
    2. move into the wheelie position
    3. perform turns while holding the wheelie position
    4. statically hold the wheelie position after being placed in it by the therapist

147. A physical therapist works on a rehabilitation unit with a physical therapist assistant. Which of the following activities would not be appropriate for a physical therapist assistant to perform?

    1. application of superficial modalities
    2. instruction of a patient in gait training
    3. document patient care activities in the medical record
    4. modification of an established plan of care

148. A patient sustains a traction injury to the brachial plexus in a motor vehicle accident and has resultant C5 and C6 nerve root involvement. Which of the following muscles would be most affected by the injury?

    1. flexor carpi ulnaris
    2. levator scapulae
    3. pectoralis minor
    4. pectoralis major

149. A physical therapist observes a burn on the dorsal surface of a patient's arm. The therapist notes that the wound appears to involve the epidermis and most of the dermis. The wound area is mottled red with a number of blisters. The therapist informs the patient that healing should take place in less than three weeks. This description is most indicative of a:

    1. superficial burn
    2. superficial partial-thickness burn
    3. deep partial-thickness burn
    4. full-thickness burn

150. A group of physical therapists develops a research project that examines the effect of increased abdominal muscle strength on forced vital capacity and forced expiratory volume. In order to conduct the study, the therapists are required to have the approval of the Hospital Institutional Review Board. The primary purpose of the committee is to:

    1. protect the hospital from unnecessary litigation
    2. ensure that established patient care standards are not compromised
    3. examine the design of the research project
    4. assess the financial ramifications of the research project

151. Members of a community health task force evaluate a proposal for a new adolescent screening program. Several members of the task force raise questions as to the validity of the screening instrument. Which measure of validity examines the instrument's ability to identify diseased persons by comparing true positives?

    1. adaptability
    2. selectivity
    3. sensitivity
    4. specificity

152. A patient who has difficulty controlling the release and retention of urine uses a urinary catheter. Upon beginning an examination, the physical therapist notices that the collection bag is almost completely full. The most appropriate action is to:

    1. continue with the examination and periodically monitor the collection bag
    2. disconnect the collection bag during the examination
    3. empty the collection bag
    4. contact the patient's nurse and request assistance

153. A physical therapist discusses the importance of proper skin care with a patient and his family. Which of the following sites is least likely to develop a pressure ulcer in a patient that is wheelchair dependent?

    1. scapula
    2. ischium
    3. heel
    4. elbow

154. A group of physical therapists conducts scoliosis screenings on adolescents as part of physical therapy week. The most appropriate action after identifying an adolescent with a moderate scoliotic curve is to:

    1. refer the adolescent for further orthopedic assessment
    2. educate the adolescent as to the cause of the scoliosis
    3. devise an exercise program for the adolescent
    4. instruct the adolescent in the importance of proper posture

155. A physical therapist orders a wheelchair for a patient recently admitted to a rehabilitation hospital. How many inches above the chair seat is the armrest on a standard adult wheelchair?

   1. 5 inches
   2. 7 inches
   3. 9 inches
   4. 11 inches

156. A physical therapist designs a treatment program for a patient with a traumatic brain injury. The patient currently is classified as confused-agitated using the Rancho Los Amigos Levels of Cognitive Functioning Scale. Which of the following guidelines would be the least beneficial when developing the treatment program?

   1. The therapist should emphasize previously learned skills and avoid teaching only new skills.
   2. The therapist should maintain a calm and focused affect.
   3. The therapist should concentrate on one specific activity for each treatment session.
   4. The therapist should schedule the patient at the same time and same place each day.

157. A physical therapist orders a wheelchair for a patient with C7 complete tetraplegia. Which of the following wheelchairs would be the most appropriate for the patient?

   1. electric wheelchair with chin controls
   2. manual wheelchair with handrim projections
   3. manual wheelchair with friction surface handrims
   4. manual wheelchair with standard handrims

158. A physical therapist checks the water temperature of the hot pack machine after several patients report the heat being very strong. Which of the following temperatures would be acceptable?

   1. 71 degrees Celsius
   2. 88 degrees Celsius
   3. 130 degrees Fahrenheit
   4. 190 degrees Fahrenheit

The following information should be used to answer questions 159 and 160:

A physical therapist examines a 22-year-old female athlete who sustained an ankle sprain three days ago playing soccer. The patient is currently full weight bearing, however walks with an antalgic gait. In order to assess the ligamentous integrity of the ankle, the therapist prepares to administer the anterior drawer test. The therapist positions the patient in supine and stabilizes the tibia and fibula.

159. The most appropriate method for performing the anterior drawer test is:

1. maintain the foot in neutral and draw the talus forward
2. maintain the foot in 20 degrees of plantar flexion and draw the talus forward
3. maintain the foot in neutral and draw the calcaneus forward
4. maintain the foot in 20 degrees of plantar flexion and draw the calcaneus forward

160. A positive anterior drawer test would be, at the very least, indicative of:

1. disruption to the anterior talofibular ligament
2. disruption to the calcaneofibular ligament
3. disruption to the anterior talofibular ligament, and calcaneofibular ligament
4. disruption of the anterior talofibular ligament, calcaneofibular ligament, and deltoid ligament

161. A physical therapist employed in an outpatient physical therapy clinic attempts to obtain informed consent from a 17-year-old male prior to initiating a formal exercise test. The patient signs the informed consent form, however the patient's parents dropped him off at the clinic and are now unavailable to sign the form. The most appropriate therapist action is:

1. complete the exercise test
2. secure another physical therapist to witness the exercise test
3. contact the referring physician and request approval to complete the exercise test
4. reschedule the exercise test

162. A patient who has completed six months of therapy receives a referral for eight additional weeks of physical therapy. The physical therapist feels the patient has reached a plateau and is not a realistic candidate for continued therapy. The therapist's most appropriate action is to:

    1. continue the patient in physical therapy for eight additional weeks
    2. reexamine the patient and develop new short and long-term goals
    3. conduct a four week trial to determine if the patient can make objective progress
    4. contact the referring physician and discuss the concerns regarding the patient's rehabilitation potential

163. A physical therapist attempts to assess developmental gross and fine motor skills in a pediatric population ranging from six to ten years of age. The most appropriate pediatric assessment tool is:

    1. Peabody Developmental Motor Scale
    2. Bruininks-Oseretsky Motor Development Scale
    3. Erhardt Developmental Prehension Assessment
    4. Gross Motor Function Measure

164. A physical therapist attempts to obtain a general assessment of a patient's cognitive status. The patient is a 62-year-old female three days status post total hip replacement. The most appropriate action is:

    1. review the patient's medical record
    2. conduct a patient interview
    3. conduct a physical examination
    4. consult with family members

165. A patient suffers a chemical burn on the cubital area of the elbow. Which position would be the most appropriate for splinting of the involved upper extremity?

    1. elbow flexion and forearm pronation
    2. elbow flexion and forearm supination
    3. elbow extension and forearm pronation
    4. elbow extension and forearm supination

166. Electromyography is performed on a patient to objectively determine the extent of pathology after sustaining a brachial plexus injury. Which of the following responses is most indicative of a normal muscle at rest?

    1. electrical silence
    2. spontaneous potentials
    3. polyphasic potentials
    4. occasional motor unit potentials

167. A patient with a C7 nerve root injury is examined in physical therapy. Which of the following objective findings would be most indicative of C7 involvement?

    1. paresthesia over the little finger
    2. weak triceps and wrist flexor muscles
    3. paresthesia over the thumb
    4. weak biceps and supinator muscles

168. A physical therapist examines a patient diagnosed with acromioclavicular joint dysfunction. The therapist instructs the patient to abduct his arm in a coronal plane to 180 degrees. Which portion of the range of motion would you most expect to elicit pain in the acromioclavicular joint?

    1. 30-70 degrees
    2. 50-90 degrees
    3. 90-120 degrees
    4. 120-180 degrees

169. A physical therapist employed in a skilled nursing facility frequently treats cognitively impaired elderly patients. Which of the following guidelines is not recommended when working with this particular population?

    1. encourage the use of hands on treatment
    2. explain frequently, consistently, and repetitively when necessary
    3. change the patient's environment and staff frequently
    4. simplify commands and label items for easy recognition

170. A physical therapist completes a quantitative gait analysis on a patient rehabilitating from a lower extremity injury. As part of the examination the therapist measures the number of steps taken by the patient in a 30 second period. This measurement technique can be used to measure:

1. acceleration
2. cadence
3. velocity
4. speed

171. Members of a health promotion task force design a program that annually will screen individuals in selected retirement communities for osteoporosis. Which screening tool would be the most cost effective and reliable to incorporate as part of the program?

1. physical activity survey
2. dietary analysis
3. measuring height
4. urinalysis screening

172. A cardiac patient undergoes a low-level symptom limited exercise treadmill test that begins at 1.5 METs and progresses to 4 METs. Which of the following activities would require an energy expenditure of approximately 4 METs?

1. sitting quietly at rest
2. level walking at 1 mph
3. level walking at 3 mph
4. level walking at 5 mph

173. A physical therapist prepares a patient for prosthetic training. Which of the following amputations would require the highest energy expenditure when using the appropriate prosthesis?

1. bilateral transtibial amputations
2. unilateral transtibial amputation
3. unilateral transfemoral amputation
4. Syme's amputation

174. A patient rehabilitating from a total hip replacement is scheduled for home physical therapy. The physical therapist assigned to the case attempts to schedule the patient, but the patient indicates that she will be unavailable for the next week due to a death in the family. The most appropriate therapist action is to:

1. insist that the patient participate in physical therapy
2. discharge the patient secondary to noncompliance
3. document the conversation with the patient and notify the physician
4. ask the physician to convince the patient to begin physical therapy immediately

175. A physical therapist positions a patient in prone with the knee flexed to 70 degrees prior to completing a manual muscle test of the hamstrings. To isolate the biceps femoris the therapist should:

1. place the thigh in slight lateral rotation and the lower leg in slight lateral rotation on the thigh
2. place the thigh in slight medial rotation and the lower leg in slight medial rotation on the thigh
3. position the knee in 90 degrees of flexion
4. position the knee in 110 degrees of flexion

176. A physical therapist reviews a patient's blood gas analysis. The therapist identifies that the $PaCO_2$ is elevated and the pH is below the normal level. These findings are most representative of:

1. respiratory acidosis
2. respiratory alkalosis
3. metabolic acidosis
4. metabolic alkalosis

177. A physical therapist strongly suspects a patient is intoxicated after arriving for his treatment session. When asked if he has been drinking, the patient indicates he consumed six or seven alcoholic beverages before driving to therapy. The therapist's most appropriate action is to:

1. continue to treat the patient, assuming he can remain inoffensive to other patients
2. modify the patient's present treatment program to minimize the effects of alcohol
3. contact a member of the patient's family to take the patient home
4. instruct the patient to leave the clinic

178. A physical therapist instructs a patient to complete a biceps strengthening exercise using a ten pound dumbbell in standing. The exercise requires the patient to maximally flex her elbow twelve times without moving the trunk. While observing the patient performing the exercise, it becomes apparent that the patient is unable to maintain her trunk in a stationary position. Which of the following modifications would be the most appropriate?

1. decrease the number of repetitions to six
2. decrease the dumbbell weight to five pounds
3. instruct the patient to perform the exercise while sitting on a stool
4. no modifications is necessary

179. A physical therapist prepares to apply a sterile dressing to a wound after debridement. The therapist begins the process by drying the wound using a towel. The therapist applies medication to the wound using a gauze pad and then applies a series of dressings that are secured using a bandage. Which step would not warrant the use of sterile technique?

1. bandage
2. dressings
3. medication
4. towel

180. A physical therapist interviews a patient in an attempt to gather information to assist with discharge planning. The patient is rehabilitating from an intertrochanteric fracture sustained six weeks ago after a fall. The patient has moderate dementia, but has no other significant past medical history. Which of the following situations would present the patient with the largest barrier toward living independently?

1. The patient resides alone and has no outside support from family or friends.
2. The patient is no longer able to drive and relies on a neighbor for all cooking, cleaning, and shopping.
3. The patient has a two story home.
4. The patient resides with a woman who has rheumatoid arthritis.

181. A physical therapist examines a patient diagnosed with Guillain-Barre syndrome. Which of the following signs or symptoms is not typically associated with this condition?

    1. difficulty breathing
    2. areflexia
    3. weakness
    4. absent sensation

182. A 78-year-old male, one month status post open reduction and internal fixation of an intertrochanteric fracture is referred to physical therapy. The patient has pain with active movement and decreased hip range of motion. Which of the following modalities would be contraindicated for the patient?

    1. moist heat
    2. pulsed ultrasound
    3. cryotherapy
    4. shortwave diathermy

183. A physical therapist examines a 42-year-old self referred female. The patient describes the onset of a variety of medical problems approximately one month ago. The patient's reported problems include right lower extremity weakness, decreased balance, and blurred vision. The physical therapy examination confirms the patient's complaints, in addition to identifying decreased pinprick sensation and ankle clonus in the right lower extremity. The most likely diagnosis is:

    1. diabetes
    2. multiple sclerosis
    3. CVA
    4. Parkinson's disease

184. A physical therapist performs a wheelchair evaluation for a patient with multiple sclerosis. The patient recently fell while ambulating and sustained a fracture of the right tibia. Since the patient is presently unable to bear weight through the involved extremity, the patient has difficulty transferring from a chair to a bed. Which of the following wheelchair prescriptions is most appropriate for the patient?

    1. light weight wheelchair, removable armrests, removable elevating leg rests
    2. light weight wheelchair, removable armrests, nonremovable leg rests
    3. light weight wheelchair, nonremovable armrests, removable elevating leg rests
    4. standard wheelchair, nonremovable armrests, and leg rests

185. A physical therapist positions a patient in sidelying and performs a talar tilt test. A positive talar tilt test would be most indicative of a:

1. calcaneofibular ligament injury
2. posterior talofibular ligament injury
3. deltoid ligament injury
4. excessive tibial torsion

186. A physical therapist listens to the lung sounds of a 56-year-old male with chronic bronchitis. The patient was admitted to the hospital two days ago after complaining of shortness of breath and difficulty breathing. While performing auscultation the therapist identifies distinct lung sounds with a relatively high constant pitch during exhalation. This type of sound is most consistent with:

1. crackles
2. rales
3. rhonchi
4. wheezes

187. A physical therapist administers iontophoresis to a patient with a lower extremity injury in an attempt to decrease the patient's soft tissue pain through the use of a local anesthetic. Which pharmacological agent would best meet the stated objective?

1. acetic acid
2. dexamethasone
3. lidocaine
4. zinc oxide

188. A physical therapist completes a daily progress note utilizing a S.O.A.P. format. Which of the following entries would not belong in the objective section?

1. will receive continuous ultrasound to the right anterior shoulder at 1.5 W/cm^2 for 5 minutes
2. incision on the left anterior forearm covered with steri-strips
3. left lower extremity range of motion within normal limits
4. tenderness to palpation in L1-L2 area

189. A physical therapist treats a patient with Parkinson's disease. The patient has trouble initiating movement and is unable to ambulate independently. The patient reports that he has fallen on three separate occasions within the last two months while attempting to ambulate. Which assistive device would be the most appropriate for the patient?

1. rolling walker
2. walker
3. axillary crutches
4. small base quad cane

190. A patient with muscle weakness and compromised balance uses a four-point gait pattern with two canes. When ascending stairs the most practical method is to:

1. use the handrail with the right hand and place the two canes in the left hand
2. use the handrail with the left hand and place the two canes in the right hand
3. place one cane in each hand and avoid using the handrail
4. place the two canes in the left hand and avoid using the handrail

191. A physical therapist receives a referral for a patient who is one week status post head injury. In the patient's medical record it notes that the patient demonstrates decorticate posturing. This type of posturing is characterized by:

1. upper extremity extension and lower extremity flexion
2. upper extremity flexion and lower extremity flexion
3. upper extremity extension and lower extremity extension
4. upper extremity flexion and lower extremity extension

192. A twelve-month-old child with cerebral palsy demonstrates an abnormal persistence of the positive support reflex. During therapy this would most likely interfere with:

1. sitting activities
2. standing activities
3. prone on elbows activities
4. supine activities

193. A physical therapist treats a patient with limited shoulder range of motion. The therapist hypothesizes that the patient's range of motion limitation is due to pain and not a specific tissue restriction. Which mobilization grades would be most appropriate to treat this patient?

    1. Grades I, II
    2. Grades II, III
    3. Grades III, IV
    4. Grades IV, V

194. A physical therapist assesses the hip range of motion of a patient with excessive anteversion. Which of the following clinical findings is common in a patient with anteversion?

    1. increased hip lateral rotation and decreased medial rotation
    2. increased hip medial rotation and decreased lateral rotation
    3. increased hip abduction and decreased adduction
    4. increased hip flexion and decreased extension

195. A patient diagnosed with lateral epicondylitis is referred to physical therapy. The therapist elects to use iontophoresis over the lateral epicondyle. Which type of current would the physical therapist use to administer the treatment?

    1. direct
    2. alternating
    3. pulsatile
    4. interferential

196. A patient with hemiplegia ambulates with an ankle-foot orthosis. The physical therapist notes that the patient's involved foot frequently drags during the initial swing phase of gait. To treat this problem most effectively the therapist should emphasize:

    1. eccentric strengthening of the hamstrings
    2. eccentric strengthening of the gluteus medius
    3. concentric strengthening of the plantar flexors
    4. concentric strengthening of the iliopsoas/rectus femoris

197. A physical therapist using the upper extremity D1 extension proprioceptive neuromuscular facilitation pattern resists elbow extension with the goal of increasing the patient's ability to extend her wrist. This is an example of:

    1. reciprocal excitation
    2. successive induction
    3. irradiation
    4. quick stretch

198. A patient who has suffered a CVA four weeks ago is beginning to show the ability to produce movement patterns outside of limb synergies. According to Brunnstrom, this patient is in which stage of recovery?

    1. two
    2. three
    3. four
    4. six

199. A physical therapist works with a patient to improve bed mobility. Which of the following techniques would be the most effective to increase the patient's hip stability?

    1. lower trunk rotation in the hooklying position
    2. bridging
    3. assisted hip and knee flexion in supine
    4. hip abduction and adduction in the hooklying position

200. A physical therapist completes a posture screening and a gross range of motion test on a patient referred to therapy with patella tendonitis. The therapist determines that the patient has extremely limited lower extremity flexibility, most notably in the hip flexors. What common structural deformity is often associated with tight hip flexors?

    1. scoliosis
    2. kyphosis
    3. lordosis
    4. spondylosis

Answer Key

1. Answer: 1   Resource: Minor (p. 309)
   When ascending a curb a patient should lead with the uninvolved lower extremity in order to avoid placing unnecessary force on the involved extremity.

2. Answer: 2   Resource: Pierson (p. 133)
   A hydraulic lift can be a safe and efficient mode to transfer large or dependent patients with little physical exertion.

3. Answer: 2   Resource: Magee (p. 225)
   Passive shoulder complex abduction is approximately 180 degrees, however glenohumeral abduction is 120 degrees with approximately 60 degrees of motion occurring at the scapulothoracic articulation.

4. Answer: 1   Resource: Kendall (p. 147)
   Individuals with weakness of the abdominal muscles often present with an anterior pelvic tilt and thus a lordotic posture or "sway-back."

5. Answer: 4   Resource: Pierson (p. 61)
   As the intensity of exercise plateaus, a patient will accommodate to the level of exercise and his/her respiration rate will tend to decrease.

6. Answer: 1   Resource: Brannon (p. 50)
   Vital capacity is defined as the amount of air that can be exhaled following a maximal inspiratory effort. Vital capacity varies directly with height and indirectly with age.

7. Answer: 1   Resource: Kendall (p. 385)
   The infraspinatus muscle is innervated by the suprascapular nerve (C4, C5, C6) which extends from the superior trunk of the brachial plexus.

8. Answer: 3   Resource: Paz (p. 616)
   Repositioning the bedrail is an immediate and appropriate response that is within the therapist's scope of practice.

9. Answer: 2   Resource: American College of Sports Medicine (p. 145)
   The American College of Sports Medicine recommends prescribing the intensity of exercise as 60 to 90% of maximum heart rate or 50-85% of $VO_{2\,max}$ or heart rate reserve.

10. Answer: 4   Resource: Minor (p. 54)
    Once a nonsterile object is placed within a sterile field, the entire sterile field should be considered nonsterile.

11. Answer: 3   Resource: Norkin (p. 26)
Although the patient can flex his right shoulder to 173 degrees, the information provided in the question did not indicate whether the starting position was equal to 0. Documentation must specify whether the range of motion was active or passive.

12. Answer: 3   Resource: Rothstein (p. 995)
Protective asepsis for respiratory isolation includes a mask. Examples of conditions that may require respiratory isolation include measles, mumps, and pertussis.

13. Answer: 4   Resource: Pauls (p. 421)
Athetosis refers to involuntary movements characterized as slow, irregular, and twisting. This type of motor disturbance makes it extremely difficult to maintain a static body position.

14. Answer: 2   Resource: Bickley (p. 600)
Wernicke's aphasia refers to an inability to comprehend written or spoken words. As a result of this condition it is inappropriate to provide detailed instructions.

15. Answer: 2   Resource: Guide for Professional
                                                        Conduct
Determining weight bearing status is the responsibility of the referring physician.

16. Answer: 3   Resource: Pierson (p. 314)
Although it is strongly recommended that healthcare employees receive the hepatitis B vaccine, it is not mandated by O.S.H.A.

17. Answer: 1   Resource: Minor (p. 290)
The parallel bars, without the use of another assistive device, provide the most stable setting for the patient to begin ambulation activities. The setting is often ideal for patients who appear to be anxious or apprehensive.

18. Answer: 4   Resource: Pierson (p. 193)
A walker with a platform attachment will provide the stability the patient requires to maintain toe-touch weight bearing while avoiding significant pressure on the upper extremity.

19. Answer: 2   Resource: Pierson (p. 123)
A sliding board transfer is possible based on the patient's upper extremity strength. The transfer will allow the patient to maintain a high level of independence.

20. Answer: 4   Resource: Magee (p. 321)
Full extension and supination is the close packed position of the ulnohumeral joint.

21. Answer: 3   Resource: Hoppenfeld (p. 101)
The flexor digitorum profundus is responsible for flexing the distal interphalangeal joint of the four fingers and assisting with flexion of the proximal interphalangeal and metacarpophalangeal joints.

22. Answer: 1   Resource: Magee (p. 691)
The iliotibial band serves as a secondary restraint to the anterior cruciate ligament, not the posterior cruciate ligament.

23. Answer: 2   Resource: Bly (p. 63)
Rolling from prone to supine usually occurs in the fifth month, while rolling from supine to prone occurs in the sixth month.

24. Answer: 4   Resource: Campbell-Physical Therapy
                                                        (p. 961)
An Individualized Education Plan articulates the goals and objectives of special education services for a given school aged child. The plan is for a one year period.

25. Answer: 2   Resource: Michlovitz (p. 198)
A patient report of a slight burning sensation under the soundhead can be due to inadequate coupling, loosening of the crystal or hot spots due to a high beam nonuniformity ratio.

26. Answer: 4   Resource: Irwin (p. 366)
The optimal position for the superior segments of the lower lobes is described as having the patient lie on his/her abdomen with two pillows under the hips. The therapist claps over the middle back at the tip of the scapula on either side of the spine.

27. Answer: 4   Resource: Irwin (p. 5)
A phase II cardiac rehabilitation program begins with the completion of a low level treadmill test and ends with a maximal treadmill test.

28. Answer: 3   Resource: American Heart Association
                                                        (p. 37)
Positioning the patient in supine with the legs elevated would be inappropriate first aid management. This position may be warranted in a patient with hypovolemic shock.

29. Answer: 2   Resource: Ciccone (p. 36)
The kidneys are the primary site of drug excretion, while the gastrointestinal tract and lungs are secondary sites.

30. Answer: 4   Resource: Kisner (p. 699)
Bilateral straight leg raising is contraindicated for a pregnant woman due to the excessive increase in abdominal pressure and the strain on the low back.

31. Answer: 1   Resource: Michlovitz (p. 140)
Buoyancy makes the body appear to weigh less in water than it does in air and as a result patients tend to move with greater ease when immersed in water.

32. Answer: 1   Resource: Michlovitz (p. 213)
Diathermy is considered a deep heating agent while the remaining options are superficial heating agents.

33. Answer: 1   Resource: Magee (p. 364)
Boutonniere deformity is most frequently encountered in patients with rheumatoid arthritis or status post trauma. It is caused by damage to the central tendinous slip of the extensor hood.

34. Answer: 3   Resource: Brannon (p. 106)
Patients with congestive heart failure may present with breathlessness, weakness, abdominal discomfort, and edema in the lower extremities resulting from venous stasis. Since sodium serves to retain water it is often restricted in a patient's diet.

35. Answer: 4   Resource: Hilt (p. 345)
Clinical union provides the necessary bony support to terminate external fixation. Callus formation represents the first stage in which bony union occurs, however does not offer adequate support.

36. Answer: 3   Resource: Pauls (p. 74)
Ankylosing spondylitis is a form of rheumatic disease characterized by inflammation of the spine resulting in back pain. Patients with ankylosing spondylitis often exhibit postural changes such as forward head, increased thoracic kyphosis, and loss of lumbar curvature. Spinal extension exercises are a common component of a therapeutic exercise program for patients with this condition.

37. Answer: 4   Resource: Standards of Practice
It is an appropriate action to request additional physical therapy visits from a referring physician.

38. Answer: 3   Resource: Magee (p. 237)
Full shoulder medial rotation is necessary to reach the perineum.

39. Answer: 3   Resource: Pierson (p. 267)
Any change in the color or odor of urine is significant and should therefore be reported and documented. A nurse would be the most logical health care professional to initially receive this information.

40. Answer: 4   Resource: Robinson (p. 182)

An orthotic device such as the Milwaukee brace is designed to facilitate improved alignment in the developing spine and therefore should be used until spinal growth ceases.

41. Answer: 2   Resource: Ciccone (p. 360)

Dizziness, weakness, and vomiting are all symptoms of digitalis toxicity. The condition may place a patient's safety in immediate jeopardy.

42. Answer: 3   Resource: Kettenbach (p. 125)

Equipment needs and equipment ordered are typically included in the plan section of a S.O.A.P. note.

43. Answer: 2   Resource: Walters (p. 250)

Productivity is a term used to describe the efficiency of a given worker or group of workers. Although measures of quality are often examined concurrently they are not used to determine productivity.

44. Answer: 4   Resource: Magee (p. 2)

The self referred patient offers a medical history that presents several significant issues including episodes of dizziness, neck stiffness with pain at night, and a family history of cancer. Based on the history and the date of the last medical examination, the patient should be referred to a physician.

45. Answer: 3   Resource: Brannon (p. 316)

A perceived exertion scale is a subjective scale where patients rate their exercise intensity.

46. Answer: 2   Resource: Goodman – Differential
                                                         Diagnosis (p. 38)

Open-ended questions guide the discussion, but do not restrict information to categories. Closed-ended questions are more impersonal and provide a limited number of response options.

47. Answer: 3   Resource: Standards of Practice

Direct personal contact with the referring physician is necessary to plan an effective care plan for the patient.

48. Answer: 4   Resource: Magee (p. 265)

A Bankart lesion is an avulsion of the capsule and glenoid labrum from the anterior rim of the glenoid resulting from traumatic anterior dislocation of the shoulder. Since the subscapularis is placed on stretch with lateral rotation this motion is initially limited after surgery.

49. Answer: 3   Resource: Rothstein (p. 17)
According to the Americans with Disabilities Act Accessibility Guidelines the space necessary for a 180 degree turn using a wheelchair is 60 inches.

50. Answer: 3   Resource: Ellis (p. 162)
All of the listed tasks are reasonable expectations for the patient, however moving from sitting to standing would be the most difficult due to the potential limitation in right knee range of motion as well as inadequate lower extremity strength.

51. Answer: 4   Resource: Pierson (p. 293)
Due to the probability associated with incidental contact, the front of a sterile gown below waist level is considered to be nonsterile.

52. Answer: 3   Resource: Norkin (p. 72)
Stabilization should occur on the distal humerus to prevent shoulder flexion.

53. Answer: 3   Resource: Ellis (p. 15)
A supine position will ensure patient safety and allow the therapist full access to the residual limb.

54. Answer: 1   Resource: Pauls (p. 161)
Leaving the residual limb exposed to the air at all times would result in increased edema and a poorly shaped residual limb.

55. Answer: 4   Resource: Pierson (p. 267)
Positioning the collection bag on the cross brace beneath the seat will allow for it to be below the level of the bladder.

56. Answer: 1   Resource: Kisner (p. 54)
The patient's postoperative status would require a rate of motion of one to two cycles per minute. Intermittent passive range of motion at a more rapid rate may cause discomfort, guarding, or splinting.

57. Answer: 4   Resource: O'Sullivan (p. 165)
Ataxia refers to defective muscular coordination with active movement. A gross measurement of upper extremity ataxia can be assessed through a finger to nose test.

58. Answer: 2   Resource: Sullivan – Clinical Decision
                                                                  Making (p. 71)
Rhythmic initiation is a particularly effective technique to improve motor control in patients with Parkinson's disease since they often have difficulty initiating movement.

59. Answer: 4   Resource: O'Sullivan (p. 160)
Patients with cerebellar degeneration often exhibit hypotonia, not hypertonia.

60. Answer: 3   Resource: Umphred (p. 249)
Positioning in prone over a wedge allows for the facilitation of head and back extension through visual tracking and upper extremity movement during therapeutic play.

61. Answer: 2   Resource: Ratliffe (p. 26)
Head positioning is the stimulus for the symmetrical tonic neck reflex. When the head is flexed, the upper extremities flex and the lower extremities extend. When the head extends the upper extremities extend and the lower extremities flex. The reaction of the extremities would not allow the infant to maintain a quadruped position.

62. Answer: 2   Resource: Davis (p. 119)
Inappropriate behavior is unacceptable and should not be tolerated. The therapist needs to make the patient aware that her behavior is inappropriate and offensive.

63. Answer: 3   Resource: Guide for Professional
                                                   Conduct
Scheduling with another therapist will allow the patient to be seen two times per week as indicated on the referral and will accommodate the patient's schedule.

64. Answer: 2   Resource: Sultz (p. 256)
In a capitated arrangement a physician or group of physicians is paid a specific amount of money for each patient enrolled in a specified health care plan. The amount of money per patient is based on projected utilization of services.

65. Answer: 1   Resource: Umphred (p. 780)
An articulation at the ankle joint would allow the tibia to advance forward over the fixed foot. This would assist with weight shifting during the sit to stand transfer.

66. Answer: 1   Resource: Brannon (p. 3)
A maximum heart rate increase of 20 beats per minute above resting is considered a safe guideline for a patient participating in a phase I program.

67. Answer: 3   Resource: Davis (p. 88)
The response "surgery can be a very frightening thought" is an empathetic response that demonstrates respect and acknowledgement for the patient's feelings.

68. Answer: 4   Resource: Brannon (p. 206)
Anxiety, tobacco, alcohol, and caffeine consumption can all serve to precipitate premature ventricular contractions. Sodium has not been shown to have any direct correlation with PVCs.

69. Answer: 1   Resource: Robinson (p. 23)
Phase charge is represented by the area under a single phase waveform. The unit of measure is the coulomb.

70. Answer: 2   Resource: Minor (p. 302)
Guarding should occur with one hand positioned on the patient's shoulder and the other on the hip. If a gait belt is used the lower hand should grasp the gait belt with the forearm in a supinated position.

71. Answer: 4   Resource: Pierson (p. 152)
Increased pressure in the popliteal area can lead to skin irritation and circulatory compromise.

72. Answer: 2   Resource: Levangie (p. 310)
The gluteus maximus and the hamstrings function as primary hip extensors. These muscles function in an eccentric fashion when moving from standing to sitting.

73. Answer: 2   Resource: Walter (p. 244)
Quality assurance programs which focus on process explore the methods, actions, and operations used to bring about a specific result.

74. Answer: 4   Resource: Standards of Practice
The physician should be informed about the patient's lack of progress. The patient may be discharged from physical therapy or referred back to the physician.

75. Answer: 2   Resource: Paz (p. 378)
Anemia refers to a reduction in the number of circulating red blood cells. Symptoms may include pallor, cyanosis, cool skin, vertigo, weakness, headache, and general malaise.

76. Answer: 1   Resource: Standards of Practice
The question does not present enough information to determine why the patient was not at home. As a result, the physical therapist should document the missed appointment and contact the patient to reschedule.

77. Answer: 1   Resource: Kisner (p. 693)
Turning the patient slightly to the left by placing a towel under the right side of the patient's pelvis will tend to lessen the effects of uterine compression on abdominal vessels and improve cardiac output.

78. Answer: 4   Resource: Kendall (p. 284)
Muscle testing of the middle trapezius should occur with the patient in a prone position.

79. Answer: 3   Resource: Ratliffe (p. 197)
A patient with spastic diplegia often utilizes mobility strategies such as "bunny hopping" due to the lack of dissociation of the lower extremities as well as the trunk from the pelvis. These activities should be discouraged and the focus should instead be on dissociation and reciprocal movement patterns.

80. Answer: 2   Resource: Tecklin (p. 194)
For thoracic and high level lumbar lesions the parapodium provides the necessary amount of support and is optimal to assist with standing activities. The parallel bars are the most stable assistive device to initiate standing and utilize during gait training.

81. Answer: 1   Resource: Umphred (p. 220)
Premature infants do not have the benefit of a prolonged intrauterine environment that assists in the development of flexion and as a result often tend to exhibit excessive extension. Positioning programs for this population often emphasize flexion to address this objective finding.

82. Answer: 4   Resource: Michlovitz (p. 272)
Ultraviolet light combined with topical psoralens has proven to be effective in treating psoriasis.

83. Answer: 1   Resource: Robinson (p. 6)
Ampere is the standard unit of measure for current.

84. Answer: 4   Resource: Scott – Promoting Legal
                                                             Awareness (p. 65)
Although a variety of subjective and objective data are admissible in a court of law, formal documentation is often paramount.

85. Answer: 1   Resource: Pierson (p. 221)
Maintaining a position behind the patient toward the affected side provides the therapist with the best opportunity to protect the patient in the event of a fall while ascending the stairs.

86. Answer: 3   Resource: Kisner (p. 718)
Patients with chronic venous insufficiency must wear compression stockings during periods of activity such as ambulation in order to avoid venous stasis and promote return to the heart.

87. Answer: 4   Resource: O'Sullivan (p. 540)
The patient's dependence with ambulation and transfers eliminates home care as a viable option at this time.

88. Answer: 3   Resource: Irwin (p. 360)

Segmental breathing can be an effective treatment technique designed to direct activity toward selected areas of the lungs.

89. Answer: 2   Resource: Brannon (p. 260)

A decrease in systolic blood pressure of greater than 10 mm Hg or failure of systolic blood pressure to rise with an increase in work load are indications to discontinue a graded exercise test.

90. Answer: 2   Resource: Hillegass (p. 651)

The palmar aspect of the therapist's hands should be in full contact over the affected lung segment. The therapist may elect to partially or fully overlap the hands during manual vibration.

91. Answer: 2   Resource: Goodman – Pathology
                                                                       (p. 1182)

Blood glucose level is used as an indicator of carbohydrate metabolism and is commonly assessed in patients with diabetes. Normal blood glucose values range from 80-120 mg/dL. Unstable levels or levels greater than the established values may require medical intervention and could restrict participation in selected physical therapy activities.

92. Answer: 3   Resource: Goodman – Pathology
                                                                        (p. 116)

Metabolic acidosis usually results from an excess accumulation of acids in the blood. Patients with uncontrolled diabetes may be particularly susceptible to ketoacidosis which is characterized by a fruity breath odor resulting from a build up of acids. The condition warrants immediate medical intervention.

93. Answer: 2   Resource: Norkin (p. 5)

The frontal plane divides the body into front and back halves. Movements in the frontal plane occur as side to side movements such as abduction or adduction. Rotary motion in the frontal plane occurs around an anterior-posterior axis.

94. Answer: 3   Resource: Sullivan – Clinical Decision
                                                                        Making (p. 64)

Maintained pressure is an effective technique that can be used to increase range of motion by facilitating local muscle relaxation, however it is a passive technique.

95. Answer: 4   Resource: Minor (p. 34)

An irregular pulse should be taken for 60 seconds in order to achieve an accurate measurement.

96. Answer: 2   Resource: Pierson (p. 195)
The parallel bars should be adjusted to provide 15 - 25 degrees of elbow flexion with a patient in standing and holding the parallel bars six inches anterior to his/her hips.

97. Answer: 2   Resource: Hillegass (p. 650)
Postural drainage to the posterior apical segments of the upper lobes is performed with the patient in sitting, leaning over a pillow at a 30 degree angle.

98. Answer: 4   Resource: Pierson (p. 150)
Seat width = hip width + 2 inches
Seat depth = posterior buttock to the popliteal space - 2 inches

99. Answer: 4   Resource: Goodman - Pathology
                                                         (p. 357)
Anemia is defined as a reduction in the number of circulating red blood cells per cubic millimeter. Symptoms of anemia include pallor of the skin, vertigo, and general malaise. Although a patient may sense that his muscles are weak, fatigue will have a greater impact on the patient's ability to complete a formal exercise program.

100. Answer: 1   Resource: Buchanan (p. 227)
Heterotopic ossification refers to abnormal bone growth in tissue. Signs and symptoms include decreased range of motion, local swelling, and warmth. Heterotopic ossification often occurs in patients following a head injury.

101. Answer: 1   Resource: Pierson (p. 193)
A walker provides more stability than axillary crutches and is more functional than the parallel bars.

102. Answer: 3   Resource: Kettenbach (p. 72)
The problem list should summarize the significant findings from the examination. Since the problem list relates back to the subjective and objective portion of the note each entry should be described in broad terms.

103. Answer: 3   Resource: The Educator's Guide to
                                                        the ADA (p. 96)
Questions asked during interviews should only relate to the functions associated with a given job and should not probe into an applicant's past medical or social history.

104. Answer: 2   Resource: Pierson (p. 268)
External urinary catheters are applied over the shaft of the penis and are therefore inappropriate for females.

105. Answer: 2   Resource: Pierson (p. 266)
    In order to promote optimal fluid flow from an IV when ambulating, a patient
    should grasp the pole so the infusion site is at heart level.

106. Answer: 4   Resource: Pierson (p. 57)
    The width of a bladder should be approximately 40% of the circumference of the
    midpoint of the limb. Bladder width for an average size adult is 5-6 inches.

107. Answer: 2   Resource: Kettenbach (p. 8)
    Although typewritten entries in the medical record are acceptable, they are not
    required.

108. Answer: 3   Resource: Code of Ethics
    The only viable solution to meet the patient's physical need is to allow him to use
    the bathroom.

109. Answer: 3   Resource: Pierson (p. 109)
    A patient status post total hip replacement using an anterolateral surgical
    approach would be most restricted in lateral rotation. Failure to restrict lateral
    rotation may result in hip dislocation or subluxation. Hip medial rotation would
    be most restricted using a posterolateral surgical approach.

110. Answer: 3   Resource: Pierson (p. 50)
    Pulse rate is increased with anxiety or stress.

111. Answer: 3   Resource: Davis (p. 85)
    Suggesting the patient write down questions for the physician is a practical and
    realistic option that will assist her in future interactions.

112. Answer: 1   Resource: Brannon (p. 134)
    Beta blockers decrease heart rate and the force associated with myocardial
    contraction. On an electrocardiogram beta blockers may cause sinus bradycardia.

113. Answer: 3   Resource: Michlovitz (p. 99)
    Ice massage is an accessible and effective cryotherapeutic agent that is often
    incorporated into a home exercise program to reduce inflammation.

114. Answer: 4   Resource: Kisner (p. 535)
    Many individuals are able to continue to function at high levels despite a variety
    of ligamentous and meniscal injuries, therefore functional instability provides the
    most direct support for an anterior cruciate ligament reconstruction.

115. Answer: 3   Resource: Davis (p. 85)
    In order to determine if the patient's poor attendance in therapy is due to difficulty
    understanding the scheduling card, the information must be presented in a manner
    the patient can understand.

116. Answer: 1   Resource: Brannon (p. 3)
Although resting levels of heart rate and blood pressure were not provided, a heart rate of 125 beats/minute and a respiration rate of 32 breaths/minute significantly exceed typical values.

117. Answer: 1   Resource: Clark (p. 339)
TLSOs prevent thoracic flexion and are most commonly prescribed in cases of fracture or compression of the body of the lower thoracic or upper lumbar vertebrae. TLSOs are sometimes referred to as a "Jewett brace."

118. Answer: 4   Resource: Van Deusen (p. 263)
The Fugl-Meyer Assessment of Motor Performance has demonstrated good validity and reliability for assessing motor function and balance in patients with hemiplegia.

119. Answer: 1   Resource: Hoppenfeld (p. 203)
The cuboid is located on the lateral aspect of the foot immediately posterior to the styloid process of the fifth metatarsal.

120. Answer: 3   Resource: Guide for Professional Conduct
The therapist should not alter the patient's weight bearing status without prior physician approval.

121. Answer: 4   Resource: Pierson (p. 265)
A nasogastric tube is a plastic tube that enters the body through a nostril and terminates in a patient's stomach. As a result the tube is not used for obtaining venous samples.

122. Answer: 2   Resource: Minor (p. 344)
Patients using axillary crutches often lean forward on the crutches to support the body during periods of standing. This activity can lead to damage in the axillary region.

123. Answer: 2   Resource: Norkin (p. 104)
Carpometacarpal flexion occurs in a frontal plane around an anterior-posterior axis with the patient in the anatomical position.

124. Answer: 1   Resource: Ellis (p. 12)
Frequent prone positioning is important for patients with transfemoral and transtibial amputations, however patients with transfemoral amputations are more susceptible to a hip flexion contracture.

125. Answer: 2   Resource: Paz (p. 334)
     Post-polio syndrome is a term used to describe symptoms that occur years after
     the onset of poliomyelitis. The condition is believed to result as remaining motor
     units become more dysfunctional. Sensation is typically not affected by post-
     polio syndrome.

126. Answer: 2   Resource: Paz (p. 334)
     Patients with Parkinson's disease often exhibit gait abnormalities due to difficulty
     initiating movement, rigidity, absence of equilibrium responses, and diminished
     associated reactions.

127. Answer: 2   Resource: Magee (p. 386)
     Assembling small bolts, nuts, and washers are activities used in a number of
     assessment measures which examine fine motor coordination such as the Purdue
     Peg Board Test.

128. Answer: 1   Resource: Rothstein (p. 592)
     Approximate blood pressure by age: 10-years-old 90/60 mm Hg, 30-years-old
     115/75 mm Hg, 50-years-old 125/82 mm Hg, 70-years-old 135/88 mm Hg.

129. Answer: 3   Resource: Minor (p. 39)
     Age predicted maximum heart rate = 220 - age.
     Maximum heart rate = 220 - 29 = 191.

130. Answer: 4   Resource: Guide to Physical Therapist
                                             Practice (p. S32)
     The physical therapy aide is a non-licensed worker who is trained under the
     direction of a physical therapist. Aides are involved in patient related and non-
     patient related duties, however would not be responsible for implementing an
     exercise program.

131. Answer: 2   Resource: Davis (p. 87)
     "Try to utilize your own strength to complete the transfer" is a direct statement
     which should present the patient with a clear understanding of the therapist's
     objective. It also places the patient in an active instead of a passive position.

132. Answer: 3   Resource: Magee (p. 692)
     Since all patients have different degrees of ligamentous laxity it is essential to
     establish a baseline with the uninvolved extremity prior to assessing the involved
     extremity.

133. Answer: 1   Resource: Guide for Professional
                                             Conduct
     The length of the car ride makes therapy three times a week unrealistic. If
     reducing the number of therapy visits jeopardizes the outcome of care, it may be
     appropriate to find therapy services within a narrower geographic radius.

134. Answer: 1   Resource: O'Sullivan (p. 630)
Clips often provide poor anchors and can cut the skin. Safety pins are also of questionable value, however are not as dangerous as clips.

135. Answer: 1   Resource: Robinson (p. 285)
Conventional TENS utilizes a pulse rate of 50-100 pps, short pulse or phase duration, and low intensity to deliver sensory level stimulation.

136. Answer: 4   Resource: Michlovitz (p. 132)
Treatment should be discontinued when there is any sign of heat intolerance. It is important to document the incident in order to alert other possible providers to the patient's reaction and to make the incident part of the permanent medical record.

137. Answer: 4   Resource: Sullivan – Clinical
                                           Procedures (p. 100)
The modified plantigrade position requires patients to possess control of equilibrium and proprioceptive reactions. The position offers a small base of support and high center of gravity with weight bearing occurring through the lower extremities.

138. Answer: 4   Resource: Minor (p. 299)
A swing-through gait pattern relies on the same principles as a swing-to gait pattern, however allows a patient to bring the lower extremities beyond the point to which the assistive devices were advanced.

139. Answer: 1   Resource: Haggard (p. 74)
Hands on training sessions provide unique opportunities for the therapist to assess the competence of family members in a structured environment.

140. Answer: 2   Resource: Kisner (p. 550)
Patients that demonstrate an extension lag have greater passive extension than active extension. The difference in the passive and active extension range of motion is used to quantify the amount of the lag. Bony obstruction would not produce an extension lag since passive range of motion and active range of motion would be equal.

141. Answer: 2   Resource: Norkin (p. 4)
The sagittal plane divides the body into left and right halves. Motions in the sagittal plane include flexion and extension. Bilateral shoulder flexion would create the largest forward movement and would therefore provide the greatest challenge for the patient.

142. Answer: 2   Resource: Hoppenfeld (p. 279)
Shortening of the latissimus dorsi often presents as a limitation of shoulder flexion or abduction due to the muscles origin on the external lip of the iliac crest and its insertion on the intertubercular groove of the humerus.

143. Answer: 2   Resource: Arends (p. 47)

The psychomotor domain is directed toward physical activity. The six categories of objectives in the psychomotor domain according to Bloom's taxonomies are reflex movements, basic fundamental movements, perceptual abilities, physical abilities, skilled movements, and non-discursive communications.

144. Answer: 3   Resource: Pierson (p. 281)

The first and most appropriate action is to put on gloves. Although direct pressure over the laceration is necessary, a therapist must always protect him/herself first.

145. Answer: 1   Resource: Umphred (p. 492)

Self range of motion of the lower extremities is a realistic goal at the C7 spinal injury level, but not at C5.

146. Answer: 4   Resource: Buchanan (p. 139)

Holding the wheelie position after being placed into it by the therapist requires the least skill and therefore provides the patient with the opportunity to gain a sense of balance before moving on to more difficult activities.

147. Answer: 4   Resource: Guide to Physical Therapist Practice (p. S42)

A physical therapist assistant can modify a specific intervention procedure when necessitated by a change in patient status, however cannot alter an established plan of care.

148. Answer: 4   Resource: Kendall (p. 277)

The upper fibers of the pectoralis major are innervated by the lateral pectoral nerve C5, 6, 7.

149. Answer: 2   Resource: O'Sullivan (p. 848)

A superficial partial-thickness burn involves both the epidermis and a portion of the dermis. Healing typically occurs in approximately three weeks with little or no scarring.

150. Answer: 2   Resource: Currier (p. 52)

Institutional review boards are responsible for assuring the welfare and safety of patients and establishing that ethical, moral, and legal standards are not compromised by proposed research activity.

151. Answer: 3   Resource: Domholdt (p. 509)

Sensitivity is the percentage of individuals with a particular diagnosis who are correctly identified as positive by a test.

152. Answer: 4   Resource: Pierson (p. 267)

Failure to allow for adequate flow of urine into a collection bag can lead to serious medical complications. A nurse should be contacted to assist with emptying the collection bag prior to continuing the physical therapy examination.

153. Answer: 4   Resource: Pierson (p. 36)

The elbow is not typically in direct contact with a given component of a wheelchair and is therefore not likely to be the site of a pressure ulcer.

154. Answer: 1   Resource: Guide for Professional
                                                      Conduct

An adolescent with a moderate scoliotic curve should be referred to a physician for further assessment.

155. Answer: 3   Resource: Pierson (p. 149)

The armrest of the wheelchair should be approximately nine inches above the wheelchair seat. This level allows the typical user to sit upright with the shoulders level while bearing weight on the forearms positioned on the armrests.

156. Answer: 3   Resource: O'Sullivan (p. 800)

Patients in the confused-agitated stage have a short attention span and therefore require numerous activities.

157. Answer: 3   Resource: O'Sullivan (p. 898)

Friction surface handrims assist a patient without a strong grasp to propel the wheelchair.

158. Answer: 1   Resource: Michlovitz (p. 116)

Hot packs should be stored in water that is approximately 160 degrees Fahrenheit or 71 degrees Celsius.

159 Answer: 2   Resource: Magee (p. 801)

By maintaining the foot in a plantar flexed position the anterior talofibular ligament is positioned perpendicular to the long axis of the tibia.

160. Answer: 1   Resource: Magee (p. 801)

A positive anterior drawer test is indicative of a tear of the anterior talofibular ligament. When the talus is drawn forward there may be a dimple that appears over the area of the anterior talofibular ligament. Although the test is positive with isolated damage to the anterior talofibular ligament, anterior translation is greater when the damage is to both the anterior talofibular ligament and the calcaneofibular ligament.

161. Answer: 4   Resource: Scott - Professional Ethics
                                                         (p. 46)
Therapists have an obligation to obtain informed consent from patients prior to
initiating intervention activities. If a patient is under the age of 18 the therapist is
required to obtain informed consent from the patient and a parent or legal
guardian.

162. Answer: 4   Resource: Guide for Professional
                                                         Conduct
The therapist should not provide additional services when he/she believes the
patient will no longer benefit from therapy.

163. Answer: 2   Resource: Van Deusen (p. 381)
The Bruininks-Oseretsky Motor Development Scale is a standardized test of
developmental gross and fine motor skills. The test is designed to be
administered to children 4.5 - 14.5 years of age who appear to have motor
problems not related to obvious dysfunction. The test takes approximately 45
minutes to administer.

164. Answer: 2   Resource: Bickley (p. 107)
A patient interview provides a physical therapist with an opportunity to assess
patient cognition. This approach is often more appropriate than relying on a
previous entry in the medical record, particularly with a patient status post
surgery.

165. Answer: 4   Resource: O'Sullivan (p. 861)
Splinting in elbow extension and forearm supination will effectively limit
contractures and maximize functional use of the upper extremity.

166. Answer: 1   Resource: Nelson (p. 547)
The process of electromyography involves asking a patient to utilize a particular
muscle so that voluntary potentials can be recorded. There should not be any
recorded electrical activity in a muscle at rest.

167. Answer: 2   Resource: Hoppenfeld (p. 122)
C7 level: Motor - triceps, wrist flexors, finger extensors
            Sensation - middle finger
            Reflex – triceps

168. Answer: 4   Resource: Magee (p. 208)
Acromioclavicular dysfunction often results in a painful arc from 120-180 degrees
of abduction. A painful arc from 90-120 degrees may be indicative of
subacromial bursitis, calcium deposits or tendonitis of the rotator cuff muscles.

169. Answer: 3   Resource: Umphred (p. 804)
Changing the patient's environment and staff frequently may lead to greater levels of stress and cognitive dysfunction.

170. Answer: 2   Resource: Levangie (p. 445)
Cadence is defined as the number of steps taken by a person per unit of time.

171. Answer: 3   Resource: Pauls (p. 654)
Osteoporosis refers to a disease process that results in a reduction of bone mass. Screening by measuring height can provide an inexpensive method to screen for this disease.

172. Answer: 3   Resource: Brannon (p. 317)
Walking at 3 mph, bicycling at 6 mph or playing golf while pulling a walking cart are activities which require 3-4 METs.

173. Answer: 3   Resource: O'Sullivan (p. 669)
A patient walking at a comfortable pace with a transfemoral prosthesis requires nearly 50% more oxygen than normal. This value is significantly higher than the other stated options.

174. Answer: 3   Resource: Standards of Practice
It is important to document any delay in the initiation of physical therapy services and to notify the referring physician.

175. Answer: 1   Resource: Kendall (p. 209)
The test for the lateral hamstrings is described with the knee in 50-70 degrees of flexion with the thigh in slight lateral rotation and the lower leg in slight lateral rotation on the thigh. Pressure should be applied against the lower leg proximal to the ankle in the direction of knee extension.

176. Answer: 1   Resource: Irwin (p. 348)
Respiratory acidosis is caused by retention of carbon dioxide due to pulmonary insufficiency. Signs and symptoms include dizziness, tingling, and syncope.

177. Answer: 3   Resource: Guide for Professional
                                                        Conduct
The patient is likely to be intoxicated if he has consumed six or seven beers. Contacting a member of the family will prevent the possibility of the patient attempting to drive.

178. Answer: 2   Resource: Kisner (p. 97)
Reducing the weight to five pounds will allow the patient to maintain the integrity of the originally prescribed exercise, while allowing the patient to perform the exercise correctly.

179. Answer: 1   Resource: Pierson (p. 311)
A bandage is used to secure the underlying dressing and therefore does not come in direct contact with the wound.

180. Answer: 1   Resource: Anderson (p. 490)
A patient with moderate dementia cannot live independently without assistance and frequent supervision. Without adequate support the patient's safety is jeopardized.

181. Answer: 4   Resource: Pauls (p. 329)
Guillain-Barre is an acute polyneuropathy causing rapid, progressive loss of motor function. Although mild sensory loss can be evident, absent sensation is extremely rare.

182. Answer: 4   Resource: Michlovitz (p. 233)
Internal or external metal objects are contraindications for shortwave and microwave diathermy.

183. Answer: 2   Resource: Pauls (p. 337)
Multiple sclerosis is a progressive disease of the central nervous system marked by intermittent damage to the myelin sheath. Blurred vision and muscle weakness are common symptoms associated with this condition.

184. Answer: 1   Resource: Pierson (p. 159)
Removable armrests will assist the patient when transferring from a wheelchair to a bed. Elevating legrests can limit the amount of time the involved leg is in a dependent position.

185. Answer: 1   Resource: Magee (p. 802)
The talar tilt test is performed with the patient in supine with the knee flexed to 90 degrees. The foot should be maintained in a neutral position while the foot is moved from side to side into abduction and adduction. A positive test is indicated by excessive adduction and is most commonly associated with damage to the calcaneofibular ligament.

186. Answer: 4   Resource: Bickley (p. 228)
During expiration wheezes are often indicative of narrowed airways or an airway obstruction. This condition is most commonly associated with asthma or bronchitis.

187. Answer: 3   Resource: Ciccone (p. 157)
Lidocaine is a local anesthetic that can be utilized with iontophoresis. The primary treatment objective when utilizing lidocaine is to decrease pain and inflammation.

188. Answer: 1   Resource: Kettenbach (p. 125)
The word "will" denotes future tense. This entry is most appropriate in the plan section of a S.O.A.P. note.

189. Answer: 1   Resource: Minor (p. 294)
A rolling walker will provide the patient with the necessary stability to ambulate safely. The wheels will allow for a smoother more coordinated gait pattern.

190. Answer: 1   Resource: Minor (p. 308)
When ascending stairs patients should follow the normal flow of traffic. Since the patient does not have unilateral weakness it is most appropriate to ascend the stairs on the right. This necessitates holding the canes with the left hand and grasping the handrail with the right.

191. Answer: 4   Resource: Anderson (p. 482)
Decorticate posturing is characterized by abnormal flexor responses in the upper extremity and extensor responses in the lower extremities. The posture is usually indicative of a lesion at or above the upper brain stem.

192. Answer: 2   Resource: Ratliffe (p. 27)
The positive support reflex promotes extension of the lower extremities and trunk with weight bearing through the balls of the feet. The reflex normally integrates at two months of age.

193. Answer: 1   Resource: Kisner (p. 224)
Grade I or II oscillation or slow intermittent grade I or II sustained joint distraction are primarily utilized for pain.

194. Answer: 2   Resource: Magee (p. 621)
Anteversion refers to the degree of angulation of the neck of the femur. In adults the mean is 8-15 degrees. Patients with excessive anteversion often exhibit more than 60 degrees of hip medial rotation and decreased lateral rotation.

195. Answer: 1   Resource: Robinson (p. 340)
Direct current is necessary to ensure a unidirectional flow of ions.

196. Answer: 4   Resource: O'Sullivan (p. 268)
The hip is required to flex during initial swing to allow for proper clearance and advancement of the limb during gait. Normally, dorsiflexion also occurs. Without the use of the dorsiflexors the hip flexors need to be strengthened in order to attain proper clearance.

197. Answer: 3   Resource: Sullivan – Clinical Decision
                                                        Making (p. 25)
When resistance is applied against a strong component of a pattern it can result in irradiation or overflow of impulses from the stronger muscle group to the weaker muscle group.

198. Answer: 3   Resource: Brunnstrom (p. 45)
Stage four in Brunnstrom's six stages of recovery for hemiplegia is signified by the development of movement outside of synergy patterns.

199. Answer: 2   Resource: Sullivan – Clinical
                                                        Procedures (p. 71)
Bridging causes the muscles of the low back and the hip extensors to isometrically contract. This action promotes hip stability.

200. Answer: 3   Resource: Magee (p. 631)
Patients with tight hip flexors often exhibit increased lordosis. Shortness of the hip flexors is often identified in standing as lumbar lordosis or through a special test such as the Thomas test.

Appendix

Performance Analysis Summary

	Available Questions	Correct Questions	% Correct
Time Management Exercise	100		
Content Outline Exercise	100		
Sample Examination Exercise	200		
Total	400		

Time Management Diagnostic Sheet

	Day One	Day Two	Day Three	Total
CLASS				
STUDY				
INDIVIDUAL TIME				
SOCIAL TIME				
EXERCISE				
WORK				
SLEEP				
NAP				
SPECIAL APPOINTMENT				

Activity Log

	Day One	Day Two	Day Three
8:00			
9:00			
10:00			
11:00			
12:00			
1:00			
2:00			
3:00			
4:00			
5:00			
6:00			
7:00			
8:00			
9:00			

Relaxation Exercise

Periodically as indicated by your learning style, use the sample relaxation exercise to relieve your body of unwanted anxiety and stress. Each of the steps should be completed in a slow and somewhat exaggerated manner.

1. Take a deep breath and expire slowly.

2. Close your eyes tightly for 10 seconds and slowly open them.

3. Lift your shoulders towards your ears.

4. Make a tight fist and flex your elbows.

5. Squeeze your buttocks tightly and hold for 3 seconds.

6. Extend your knees and plantar flex your ankles.

7. Close your eyes tightly for 10 seconds and slowly open them.

8. Take a deep breath and expire slowly.

Resource List

American Physical Therapy Association
1111 North Fairfax Street
Alexandria, Virginia 22314
Phone: (800) 999-2782
Web site: www.apta.org
Fax on demand: (800) 399-2782

Federation of State Boards of Physical Therapy
509 Wythe Street
Alexandria, Virginia 22314
Phone: (703) 299-3100
Web site: www.fsbpt.org

Mainely Physical Therapy
P.O. Box 7242
Scarborough, Maine 04070-7242
Toll Free: (866) PTEXAMS
Phone: (207) 885-0304
Web site: www.ptexams.com
Fax: (207) 883-8377

Physical Therapy State Licensing Agencies

Alabama

Alabama Board of Physical Therapy
100 N. Union Street
Suite 627
Montgomery, AL 36130-5040

(334) 242-4064
www.pt.state.al.us

Arizona

Arizona State Board of Physical Therapy
1400 West Washington
Suite 230
Phoenix, AZ 85007

(602) 542-3095
www.ptboard.state.az.us

California

PT Board of California
1418 Howe Avenue
Suite 16
Sacramento, CA 95825

(916) 561-8200
www.ptb.ca.gov

Connecticut

Connecticut Dept of Public Health
410 Capitol Avenue
MS #12APP
Hartford, CT 06134-0308

(860) 509-7590
www.state.ct.us/dph/

Alaska

State PT & OT Board Div of Occup Licensing
333 Willoughby Avenue, 9th Floor
P.O. Box 110806
Juneau, AK 99811

(907) 465-2580
www.dced.state.ak.us/occ/pphy.htm

Arkansas

Arkansas State Board of Physical Therapy
9 Shackleford Plaza
Suite 3
Little Rock, AR 72211

(501) 228-7100
www.arptb.org

Colorado

Colorado Division of Registrations
1560 Broadway
Suite 1545
Denver, CO 80202

(303) 894-2440
www.dora.state.co.us/Physical-Therapy

Delaware

Division of Professional Regulation
861 Silver Lake Blvd.
Suite 203 Cannon Building
Dover, DE 19904-2467

(302) 744-4506
www.state.de.us/research/profreg/physical.htm

District of Columbia

DC Board of Physical Therapy
Dept of Health
825 N. Capital Street, NE, Rm 2224
Washington, DC 20002

(202) 442-4764

Georgia

Georgia Board of Physical Therapy
237 Coliseum Drive
Macon, GA 31217

(912) 207-1620
www.sos.state.ga.us/plb/pt/

Idaho

ID State Board of Medicine
1755 Westgate Drive
Suite 140
Boise, ID 83704

(208) 327-7000
www.bom.state.id.us

Indiana

Indiana Physical Therapy Committee
402 W. Washington Street
Room W041
Indianapolis, IN 46204

(317) 234-2051
www.in.gov/hpb/boards/ptc/

Florida

Dept of Health, MQA, Board of Physical Therapy
Practice
4052 Bald Cypress Way
Bin #C05
Tallahassee, FL 32399-3255

(850) 245-4373
www.doh.state.fl.us/mqa

Hawaii

Dept of Commerce & Consumer Affairs
P.O. Box 3469
Honolulu, HI 96801

(808) 586-2694

Illinois

Dept of Professional Regulation
320 West Washington
3rd Floor
Springfield, IL 62786

(217) 782-8556
www.dpr.state.il.us

Iowa

Board of Physical & Occupational Therapy
Examiners
Iowa Dept of Public Health
321 East 12th Street, 5th Floor
Des Moines, IA 50319-0075

(515) 281-4413

Kansas

KS State Board of Healing Arts
PT Examining Committee
235 S. Topeka Blvd
Topeka, KS 66603

(785) 296-7413
www.ink.org/public/boha

Louisiana

LA State Board of PT Examiners
714 E. Kaliste Saloom Road
Suite D2
Lafayette, LA 70508-3834

(337) 262-1043
www.laptboard.org

Maryland

Board of Physical Therapy Examiners
4201 Patterson Avenue #318
Baltimore, MD 21215-2299

(410) 764-4752
www.dhmh.state.md.us/bphte/

Michigan

Physical Therapy State Boards
P.O. Box 30670
Lansing, MI 48909

(517) 335-0918
www.cis.state.mi.us/bhser/home.htm

Mississippi

MS State Dept of Health Div of Licensure & Reg
Professional Licensure Rm 160
570 East Woodrow Wilson Blvd
Jackson, MS 39216

(601) 576-7262

Kentucky

Kentucky State Board of PT
9110 Leesgate Road, #6
Louisville, KY 40222-5159

(502) 327-8497
www.kbpt.state.ky.us

Maine

Board of Examiners in PT
35 State House Station
Augusta, ME 04330

(207) 624-8600
www.state.me.us/pfr/led/ledhome2.htm

Massachusetts

MA Board of Allied Health Professionals
Division of Registration
239 Causeway Street, Suite 500
Boston, MA 02114

(617) 727-3071
www.state.ma.us/reg/boards/ah

Minnesota

MN Board of Physical Therapy
2829 University Avenue, SE, #315
Minneapolis, MN 55414-3222

(612) 627-5406
www.physicaltherapy.state.mn.us

Missouri

Advisory Comm for Prof PTs & PTAs
P.O. Box 4
3605 Missouri Boulevard
Jefferson City, MO 65102

(573) 751-0098
www.ded.state.mo.us

Montana

Board of Physical Therapy Examiners
301 South Park, 4th Floor
P.O. Box 200513
Helena, MT 59620-0513

(406) 841-2369

Nevada

NV State Bd of Physical Therapy Examiners
3150 W. Sahara Ane.
Suite B-13
Las Vegas, NV 89102

(702) 876-5535

New Jersey

NJ State Board of PT
P.O. Box 45014
Newark, NJ 07101

(937) 504-6455

New York

State Board for PT
89 Washington Avenue
Education Bldg, East Mezzanine
Albany, NY 12234

(518) 474-3817
www.op.nysed.gov/pt.htm

Nebraska

Board of Physical Therapy
301 Centennial Mall
P.O. Box 94986
Lincoln, NE 68509

(402) 471-0547
www.hhs.state.ne.us/lis/lis.asp

New Hampshire

PT Governing Boad of NH
Office of Allied Health Prof
2 Industrial Park Drive
Concord, NH 03301

(603) 271-8389

New Mexico

NM Physical Therapy Board
2055 S. Pacheco
Suite 400
Santa Fe, NM 87505

(505) 476-7085
www.state.nm.us/rid/b&c/ptb

North Carolina

North Carolina Board of Physical Therapy
18 W. Colony Place #140
Durham, NC 27705

(919) 490-6393
www.ncptboard

North Dakota

ND State Examination Committee for PT
106 Eastern Avenue
Grafton, ND 58237

(701) 352-1621

Oklahoma

Bd of Med Lic & Sup
PT Advisory Committee
5104 North Francis, Suite C
Oklahoma City, OK 73118

(405) 848-6841
www.osbmls.state.ok.us

Pennsylvania

PA State Board of PT
P.O. Box 2649
Harrisburg, PA 17105

(717) 783-7134
www.dos.state.pa.us

Rhode Island

Rhode Island PT Board
Division of Prof Regulation
3 Capitol Hill, Room 104
Providence, RI 02908-5097

(401) 222-2827
www.health.state.ri.us

South Dakota

SD Board of Medical Examiners
1323 S. Minnesota Avenue
Sioux Falls, SD 57105

(605) 334-8343

Ohio

Ohio State Board of Physical and Occupational
Therapy
77 S. High Street
16th Floor
Columbus, OH 43215-6108

(614) 466-3774
www.state.oh.us/pyt

Oregon

PT Licensing Board
800 NE Oregon Street
Suite 407
Portland, OR 97232

(503) 731-4047
www.ptboard.state.or.us

Puerto Rico

Office of Regulation and Certification
Call Box 10200
Santurce, PR 00908

(787) 725-8161 x209

South Carolina

Board of PT Examiners
110 Centerview Drive
P.O. Box 11329
Columbia, SC 29211

(803) 896-4655
www.llr.state.sc.us

Tennessee

Div of Health Related Boards
Bd of Occupational & Physical Therapy
426 5th Ave North, 1st Floor
Nashville, TN 37247

(615) 532-5136
www.state.tn.us/health/links.html

Texas

TX Board of PT Examiners
1308 Queenspark
Austin, TX 78701

(903) 531-4330
www.ecptote.state.tx.us

Vermont

Physical Therapy Advisors
Office of Professional Regulations
26 Terrace Street, Drawer 09
Montpelier, VT 05609-1106

(802) 828-2390
www.sec.state.vt.us

Virginia

Board of Physical Therapy
Dept of Health Professions, 5th Floor
6603 West Broad Street
Richmond , VA 23230

(804) 662-9924

West Virginia

WV Board of Physical Therapy
153 W. Main Street
Suite 103
Clarksburg, WV 26301

(304) 627-2251

Wyoming

WY Board of Physical Therapy
2020 Carey Avenue
Suite 201
Cheyenne, WY   82002

(307) 777-3507

Utah

Division of Professional Licensing
160 East 300 South
Salt Lake City, UT 84114

(801) 530-6632

Virgin Islands

VI Board of PT Examiners
48 Sugar Estate
St. Thomas, VI 00802

(340) 774-0117

Washington

Washington Bd of PT
1112 SE Quince Street
P.O. Box 47868
Olympia, WA 98504-7868

(360) 236-4700
www.doh.wa.gov/hsqa/hpqad/physical_ther

Wisconsin

WI Dept of Regulation & Licensing
Rm 178, 1400 E. Washington Avenue
P.O. Box 8935
Madison, WI 53708-8935

(608) 266-2112

Prometric Testing Centers

Alaska
Anchorage

Alabama
Birmingham
Decatur
Dothan
Mobile
Montgomery

Arkansas
Arkadelphia
Fort Smith
Little Rock

Arizona
Goodyear
Phoenix
Tucson

California
Anaheim
Atascadero
Brea\Fullerton
Culver City (3)
Diamond Bar
Fair Oaks
Fremont
Gardena
Glendale (2)
Irvine
La Mesa
Palm Desert
Piedmont
Rancho Cucamonga
Redlands
Riverside
San Diego
San Francisco (2)
San Jose (2)
Santa Rosa
Walnut Creek
Westlake Village

Colorado
Boulder
Colorado Springs
Denver
Glendale
Pueblo

Connecticut
Glastonbury
Hamden
Norwalk

District of Columbia
Washington, D.C.

Delaware
Dover
Wilmington

Florida
Cassellberry
Fort Myers
Gainesville
Hollywood
Jacksonville
Maitland
Miami Lakes
Sarasota (2)
Tallahassee
Tampa
Temple Terrace

Georgia
Albany
Atlanta (2)
Augusta
Jonesboro
Macon
Savannah
Marietta (2)
Valdosta

Hawaii
Honolulu (temp)
Kailua

Iowa
Ames
Bettendorf
Sioux City
West Des Moines

Idaho
Boise

Illinois
Carbondale
Chicago (3)
Homewood
Lombard
Northbrook
Peoria
Springfield
Sycamore
Westchester

Indiana
Evansville
Fort Wayne
Indianapolis (2)
Lafayette
Merrillville
Mishawaka
Terre Haute

Kansas
Topeka
Wichita

Kentucky
Lexington
Louisville

Louisiana
Baton Rouge
Bossier City
New Orleans

Massachusetts
Boston (2)
Braintree
Brookline
East Longmeadow
Lexington
Waltham (2)
Worcester (2)

Maryland
Baltimore
Bethesda
Columbia
Lanham
Pikesville
Salisbury

Maine
Orono
South Portland

Michigan
Detroit\Southfield
Grand Rapids
Lansing
Livonia
Portage
Troy
Utica

Minnesota
Bloomington (3)
Duluth
Rochester
St. Cloud
Woodbury

Missouri
Ballwin
Cape Girardeau
Jefferson City

Lee's Summit
Springfield
St. Joseph
St. Louis

Mississippi
Jackson
Tupelo

Montana
Billings
Helena

North Carolina
Asheville
Charlotte
Gastonia
Greensboro
Greenville
Raleigh (2)
Salisbury
Wilmington

North Dakota
Bismark
Fargo

Nebraska
Columbus
Lincoln
Omaha

New Hampshire
Portsmouth

New Jersey
Deptford
East Brunswick
Fair Lawn
Toms River
Hamilton
Union (2)
Verona

New Mexico
Albuquerque

Nevada
Las Vegas (2)
Reno

New York
Albany
Amherst
Brooklyn Heights (2)
East Syracuse
Garden City
Ithaca
Melville (2)
Manhasset
Midtown (3)
New York City
Penn Plaza (3)
Queens/Rego Park
Rochester
Staten Island
Vestal
Wappingers Falls
Watertown
White Plains

Ohio
Akron
Centerville
Cincinnati (2)
Columbus
Hillard
Lima
Mentor
Niles
Reynoldsburg
Strongsville
Toledo

Oklahoma
Oklahoma City
Tulsa

Oregon
Eugene

Milwaukie
Portland

Pennsylvania
Allentown
Clarks Summit
Erie
Harrisburg
Lancaster
North Wales (2)
Philadelphia
Pittsburgh (2)
York

Rhode Island
Cranston

South Carolina
Charleston
Greenville
Myrtle Beach
Irmo

South Dakota
Sioux Falls

Tennessee
Chattanooga
Clarksville
Franklin
Knoxville
Madison
Memphis (2)

Texas
Abilene
Amarillo
Arlington
Austin
Beaumont
Bedford
Corpus Christi
El Paso
Houston
Kingwood
Lubbock
Mesquite
Midland
New Braunfels
San Antonio
Sugar Land (2)
Tyler
Waco

Utah
Odgen
Orem
Salt Lake City

Virginia
Fairfax (2)
Lynchburg
Mechanicsville
Newport News
Roanoke

Vermont
Williston

Washington
Mountlake Terrace (2)
Puyallup
Spokane

Wisconsin
Fox Point
Madison
New Berlin
Racine

West Virginia
Morgantown
S. Charleston

Wyoming
Casper

Puerto Rico
Hato Rey

Virgin Islands
St. Croix

Bibliography

American College of Sports Medicine: <u>ACSM's Guidelines for Exercise Testing and Prescription</u>, Sixth Edition, Lippincott Williams & Wilkins, 2000

American Heart Association: <u>BLS for Healthcare Providers</u>, American Heart Association, 2001

Anemaet W, Moffa-Trotter M: <u>Home Rehabilitation: Guide to Clinical Practice</u>, Mosby, Inc., 2000

Anderson D: <u>Mosby's Medical, Nursing, and Allied Health Dictionary</u>, Sixth Edition, Mosby, Inc., 2002

Arends R: <u>Learning to Teach</u>, Second Edition, McGraw-Hill, Inc., 1991

Bennett S, Karnes J: <u>Neurological Disabilities: Assessment and Treatment</u>, Lippincott-Raven Publishers, 1998

Best J, Kahn J: <u>Research in Education</u>, Fifth Edition, Prentice-Hall, 1986

Bickley L, Szilagyi P: <u>Bates' Guide to Physical Examination and History Taking</u>, Eighth Edition, Lippincott Williams & Wilkins, 2003

Bly L: <u>Motor Skill Acquisition in the First Year</u>, Therapy Skill Builders, 1994

Brannon F, Foley M, Starr J, Saul L: <u>Cardiopulmonary Rehabilitation: Basic Theory and Application</u>, F.A. Davis Company, 1998

Brunnstrom S: <u>Movement Therapy in Hemiplegia</u>, Harper and Row Publishers Inc., 1970

Buchanan L, Nawoczenski D: <u>Spinal Cord Injury: Concepts and Management Approaches</u>, Williams & Wilkins, 1987

Cameron M: <u>Physical Agents in Rehabilitation: From Research to Practice</u>, W.B. Saunders Company, 1998

Campbell S: <u>Decision Making in Pediatric Neurologic Physical Therapy</u>, Churchill Livingstone, 1999

Campbell S: <u>Physical Therapy for Children</u>, Second Edition, W.B. Saunders Company, 2000

Ciccone C: <u>Pharmacology in Rehabilitation</u>, Third Edition, F.A. Davis Company, 2002

Clark C, Bonfiglio M: Orthopaedics: Essentials of Diagnosis and Treatment, Churchill Livingstone, 1994

Code of Ethics, American Physical Therapy Association, 2001

Currier D: Elements of Research in Physical Therapy, Second Edition, Williams & Wilkins, 1984

Curtis K: The Physical Therapist's Guide to Health Care, Slack Inc., 1999

Davies P: Steps to Follow, Springer-Verlag, 1985

Davis C: Patient Practitioner Interaction, Third Edition, Slack Inc., 1998

De Domenico G, Wood E: Beard's Massage, W.B. Saunders Company, 1997

DePoy E, Gitlin L: Introduction to Research: Multiple Strategies for Health and Human Services, Mosby-Year Book, Inc., 1994

Domholdt E: Physical Therapy Research Principles and Application, Second Edition, W.B. Saunders Company, 2000

Edelman C, Mandle C: Health Promotion, Mosby, Inc., 1990

Educator's Guide to the Americans with Disabilities Act, American Vocational Association, 1993

Ellis D, Lamkowitz S, Maisey-Ireland M: Master Student, College Survival Inc., 1986

Giles S: A Guide to Success: Review for Licensure in Physical Therapy, Mainely Physical Therapy, 2002

Giles S, Stuart J: Test Master: Physical Therapist Examination, Mainely Physical Therapy, 2003

Goodman C, Boissonnault W: Pathology: Implications for the Physical Therapist, W.B. Saunders Company, 1998

Goodman C, Snyder T: Differential Diagnosis in Physical Therapy, Third Edition, W.B. Saunders Company, 2000

Goold G: First Aid in the Workplace, Prentice-Hall, 1995

Guide for Professional Conduct, American Physical Therapy Association, 2001

Guide to Physical Therapist Practice, Second Edition, American Physical Therapy Association, 2001

Haggard A: Handbook of Patient Education, Aspen Publishers, 1989

Hamill J, Knutzen K: Biomechanical Basis of Human Movement, Williams & Wilkins, 1995

Hertling D, Kessler R: Management of Common Musculoskeletal Disorders, Third Edition, Lippincott, 1996

Hillegass E, Sadowsky H: Cardiopulmonary Physical Therapy, Second Edition, W. B. Saunders, Inc., 2001

Hilt N, Cogburn S: Manual of Orthopedics, 1980

Hoppenfeld S: <u>Physical Examination of the Spine and Extremities</u>, Appleton-Century-Crofts, 1976

Irwin S, Tecklin J: <u>Cardiopulmonary Physical Therapy</u>, Third Edition, Mosby-Year Book, Inc., 1995

Kendall F, McCreary E, Provance P: <u>Muscle Testing and Function</u>, Williams & Wilkins, 1993

Kettenbach G: <u>Writing S.O.A.P. Notes</u>, Second Edition, F.A. Davis Company, 1995

Kisner C, Colby L: <u>Therapeutic Exercise Foundations and Techniques</u>, Fourth Edition, F.A. Davis Company, 2002

Levangie P, Norkin C: <u>Joint Structure and Function: A Comprehensive Analysis</u>, Third Edition, F.A. Davis Company, 2001

Magee D: <u>Orthopedic Physical Assessment</u>, Fourth Edition, W.B. Saunders Company, 2002

Michlovitz S: <u>Thermal Agents in Rehabilitation</u>, Third Edition, F.A. Davis Company, 1996

Minor M, Minor S: <u>Patient Care Skills</u>, Fourth Edition, Appleton & Lange, 1999

<u>National Physical Therapy Examinations Candidate Handbook</u>, Federation of State Boards of Physical Therapy, 2002

Nelson R, Hayes K, Currier D: <u>Clinical Electrotherapy</u>, Third Edition, Appleton & Lange, 1999

Norkin C, White D: <u>Measurement of Joint Motion: A Guide to Goniometry</u>, Edition Two, F.A. Davis Company, 1995

Nosse L, Friberg D: <u>Management Principles for Physical Therapists</u>, Williams & Wilkins, 1992

O'Sullivan S, Schmitz T: <u>Physical Rehabilitation: Assessment and Treatment</u>, Fourth Edition, F.A. Davis Company, 2001

Ozer M, Payton O, Nelson C: <u>Treatment Planning for Rehabilitation: A Patient Centered Approach</u>, McGraw-Hill, 2000

Pauls J, Reed K: <u>Quick Reference to Physical Therapy</u>, Aspen Publishers, 1996

Paz J, Panik M: <u>Acute Care Handbook for Physical Therapists</u>, Butterworth-Heinemann, 1997

<u>Physical Therapist's Clinical Companion</u>, Springhouse Corporation, 2000

Pierson F: <u>Principles and Techniques of Patient Care</u>, Second Edition, W. B. Saunders Company, 1999

Ratliffe K: <u>Clinical Pediatric Physical Therapy: A Guide for the Physical Therapy Team</u>, Mosby, Inc., 1998

Reider B: <u>The Orthopaedic Physical Examination</u>, W. B. Saunders Company, 1999

Robinson A, Snyder-Mackler L: <u>Clinical Electrophysiology</u>, Williams & Wilkins, 1995

Rothstein J, Roy S, Wolf S: <u>The Rehabilitation Specialist's Handbook</u>, F.A. Davis Company, 1998

Roy S, Irvin R: <u>Sports Medicine: Prevention, Evaluation, Management and Rehabilitation</u>, Prentice-Hall, 1983

Salter R: <u>Textbook of Disorders and Injuries of the Musculoskeletal System</u>, Third Edition, Williams & Wilkins, 1999

Scott R: <u>Health Care Malpractice: A Primer of Legal Issues for Professionals</u>, Second Edition, McGraw-Hill, Inc., 1999

Scott R: <u>Legal Aspects of Documenting Patient Care</u>, Second Edition, Aspen Publishers, Inc., 2000

Scott R: <u>Promoting Legal Awareness in Physical and Occupational Therapy</u>, Mosby, Inc., 1997

Scott R: <u>Professional Ethics: A Guide for Rehabilitation Professionals</u>, Mosby, Inc., 1998

Shamus E, Shamus J: <u>Sports Injury: Prevention & Rehabilitation</u>, McGraw-Hill Companies, Inc., 2001

Shumway-Cook A, Woollacott M: <u>Motor Control: Theory and Practical Applications</u>, Second Edition, Lippincott Williams & Wilkins, 2001

<u>Standards of Practice for Physical Therapy</u>, American Physical Therapy Association, 2002

Sullivan P, Markos P: <u>Clinical Decision Making in Therapeutic Exercise</u>, Appleton & Lange, 1995

Sullivan P, Markos P: <u>Clinical Procedures in Therapeutic Exercise</u>, Appleton and Lange, 1996

Tecklin J: <u>Pediatric Physical Therapy</u>, Edition Three, Lippincott Williams & Wilkins, 1999

Triola M: <u>Elementary Statistics</u>, Seventh Edition, Addison-Wesley Publishing Company, Inc., 1998

Trofino R: <u>Nursing Care of the Burn Injured Patient</u>, F.A. Davis Company, 1991

Umphred D: <u>Neurological Rehabilitation</u>, Fourth Edition, Mosby, Inc., 2001

Van Deusen J: <u>Assessment in Occupational and Physical Therapy</u>, W.B. Saunders, Inc., 1997

Walter J: <u>Physical Therapy Management</u>, Mosby, Inc., 1993

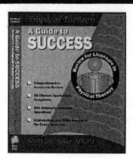
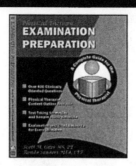
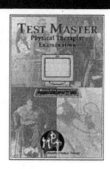